The Emotional

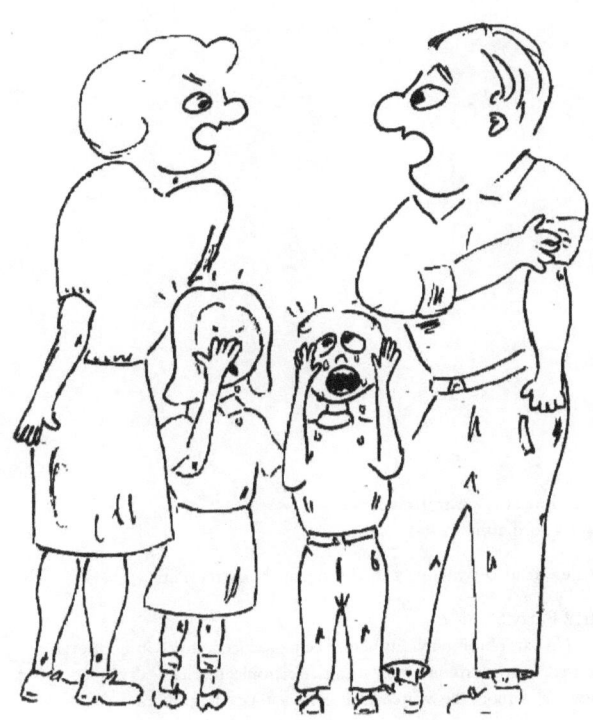

origins of
anger

Written by:
Barry Stanley
M.B., Ch.B.,F.R.C.S(C)

Illustrated by:
Ian Young

Order this book online at www.trafford.com
or email orders@trafford.com

Most Trafford titles are also available at major online book retailers.

Printed in the United States of America.

ISBN: 978-1-4669-4031-4 (sc)
ISBN: 978-1-4669-4030-7 (hc)
ISBN: 978-1-4669-4029-1 (e)

Library of Congress Control Number: 2012909832

Trafford rev. 06/19/2012

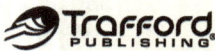 www.trafford.com

North America & International
toll-free: 1 888 232 4444 (USA & Canada)
phone: 250 383 6864 ♦ fax: 812 355 4082

THE EMOTIONAL ORIGINS OF ANGER

People who have brain injury or psychotic conditions are unable to control their anger. These notes do not apply to them.

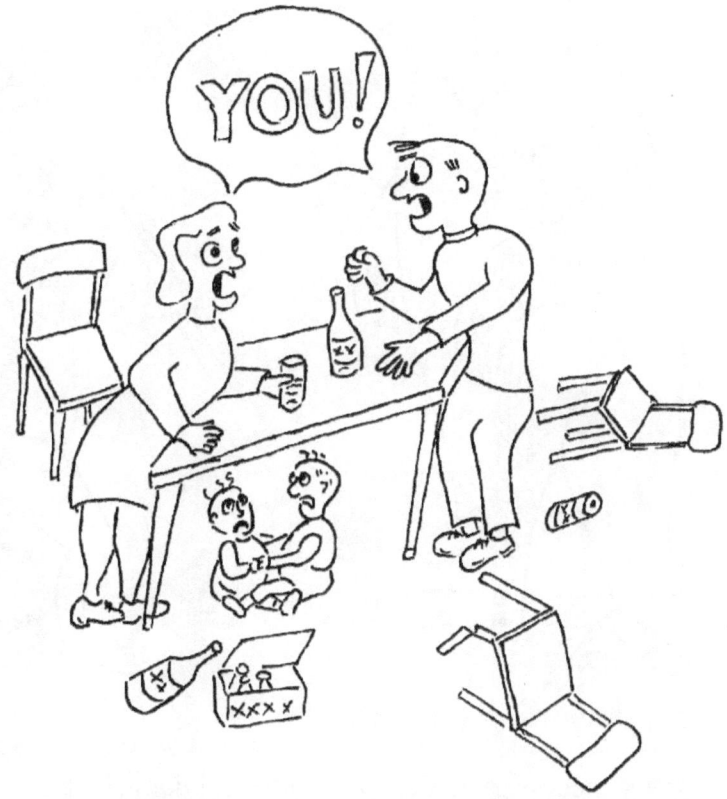

Alcohol also interferes with our ability to control our anger. Control of anger requires control of alcohol.

When we lived in caves,

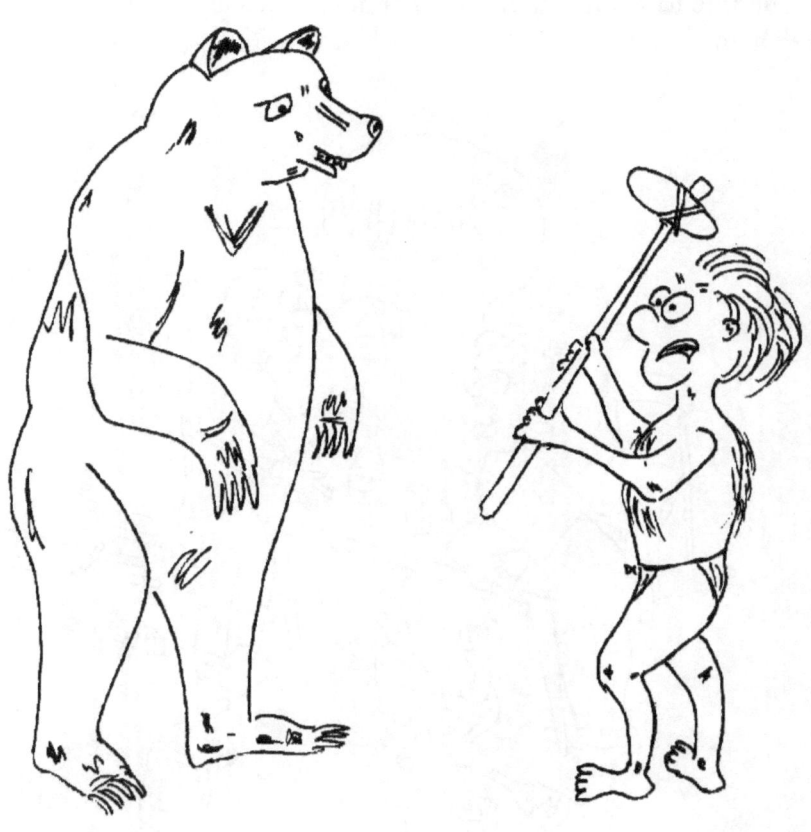

anger was necessary to deal with physical danger.

Now most of the dangers that threaten us,

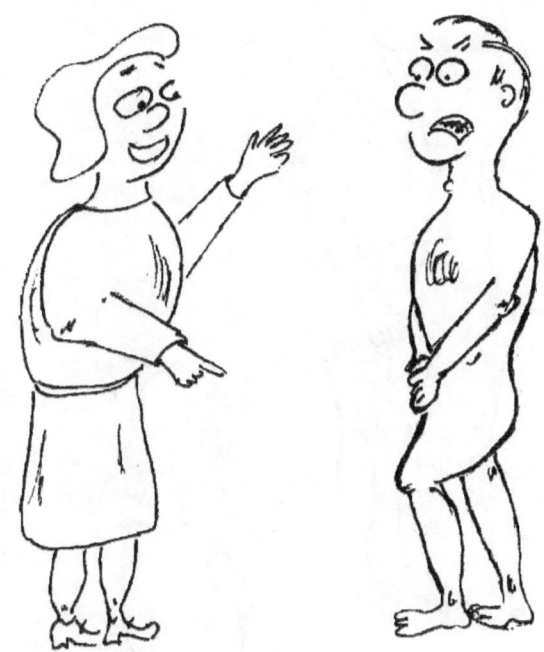

are psychological

It is no longer helpful to get angry

when we feel threatened.

Anger is a burden.

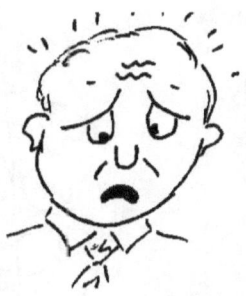

Within a few weeks of birth, a baby can show fear. It is the fundamental negative emotion, created by a real or imagined danger.

Later, the emotion of shame

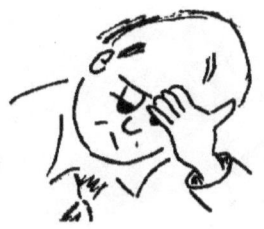

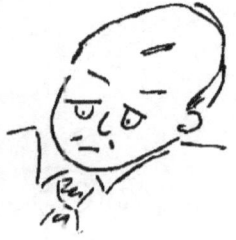

and guilt develop under the influence of the higher brain centers.

We can only experience one emotion at a time.

We cannot have two emotions simultaneously,

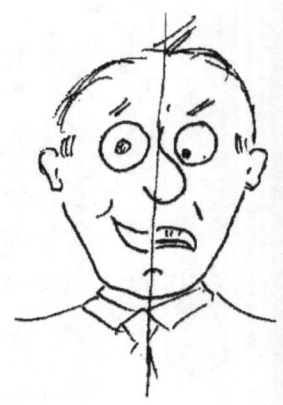

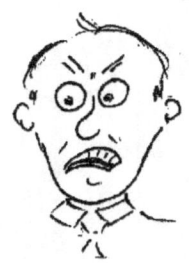

although we can go from one

to another instantaneously.

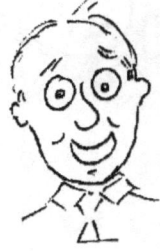

The emotion of anger is always
secondary to the emotions of

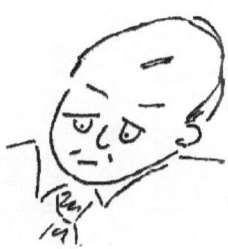

fear,

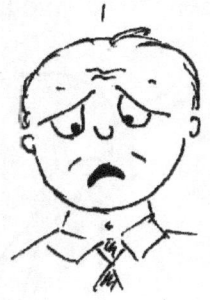

guilt,

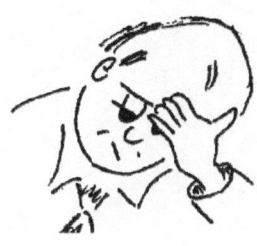

or shame.

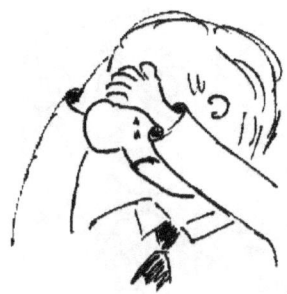

Shame is the emotion we experience when we behave in a manner that reduces our self-respect.

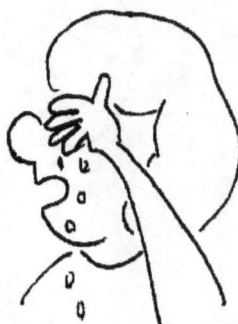

Some insecure people feel ashamed all the time about issues they are not responsible for.

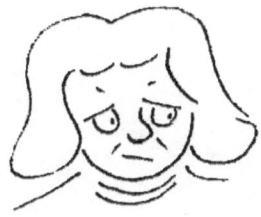

Guilt is the feeling of remorse when we acknowledge our reponsibility for the hurt we have done to others.

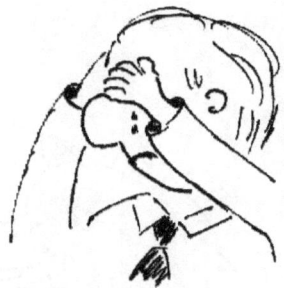

Some insecure people feel guilty all the time about issues they are not responsible for.

All other emotions

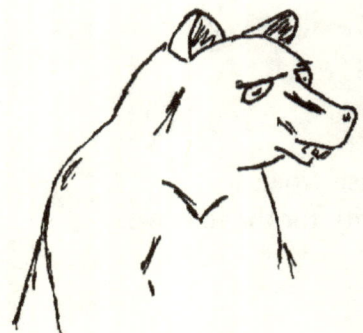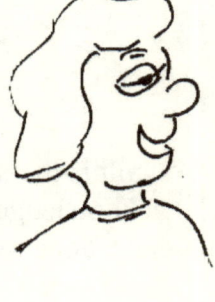

are replaced by fear

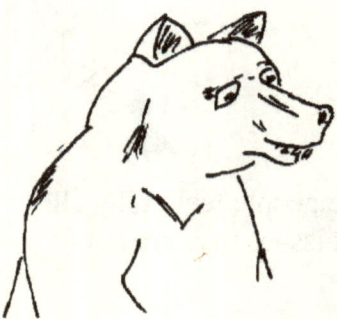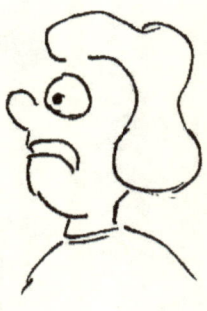

when danger threatens.

Fear is our response to anything that is a threat,

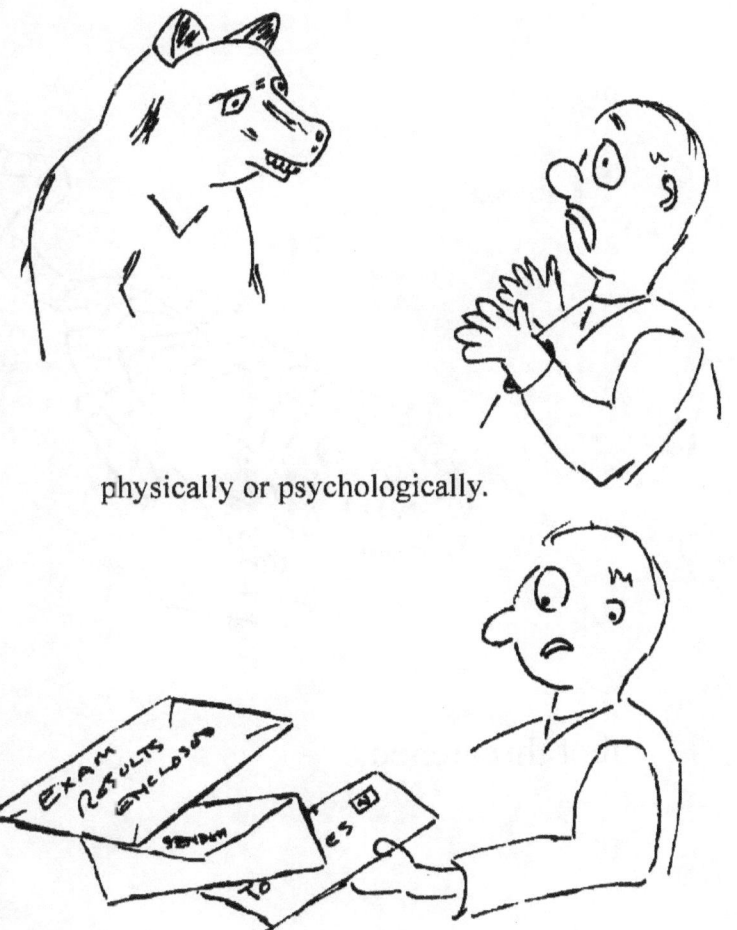

physically or psychologically.

Fear is the only emotion that is necessary for survival.
The emotion of fear is our defence mechanism against
danger.

We cannot survive without the ability to

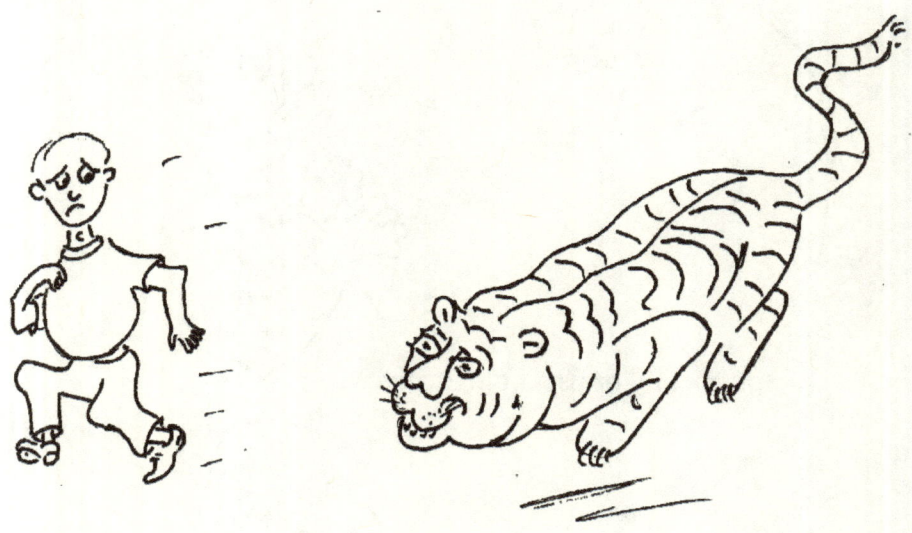

feel threatened.

If our shame,

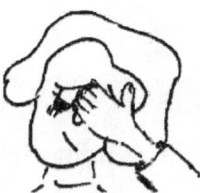

guilt

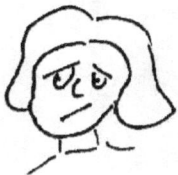

and fear

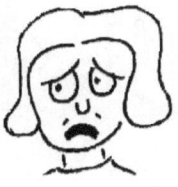

are too painful to acknowledge and deal with,

we become angry.

We do not get angry with our boss, but we may with our co-workers.

We might kick our cat

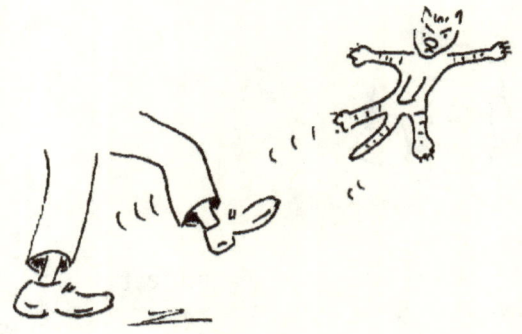

but we will never kick our pet tiger, no
matter how angry we are.

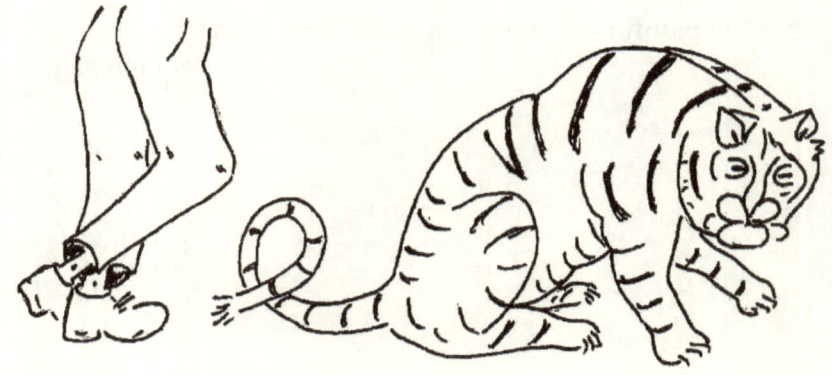

Substances, such as alcohol, interfere with our judgement. We may kick the tiger, mistaking it for the cat.

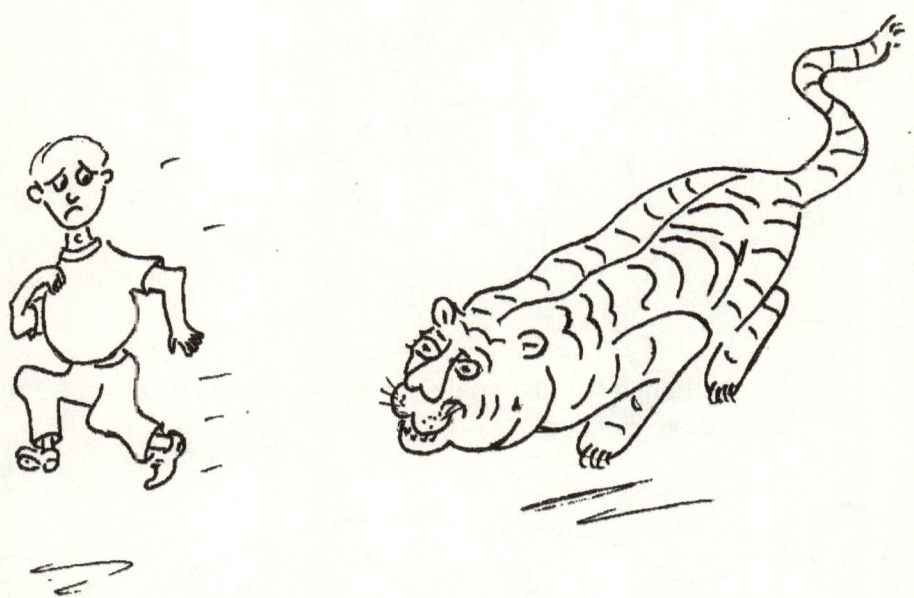

We are always making decisions about whom we can safely direct our anger towards. We are always controlling our anger. This means that we can choose not to express our anger.

We only express our anger when it is safe to do so. We only express our anger to those we perceive to be less powerful,

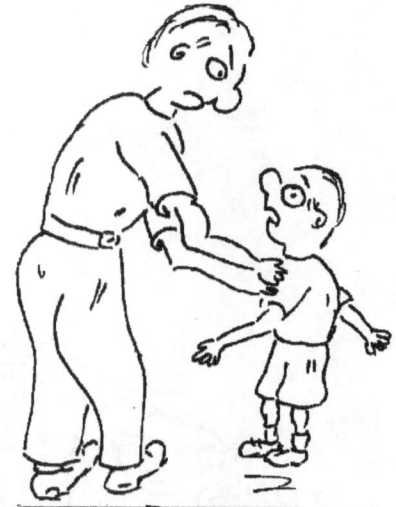

although we may make errors of judgement and suffer the consequences.

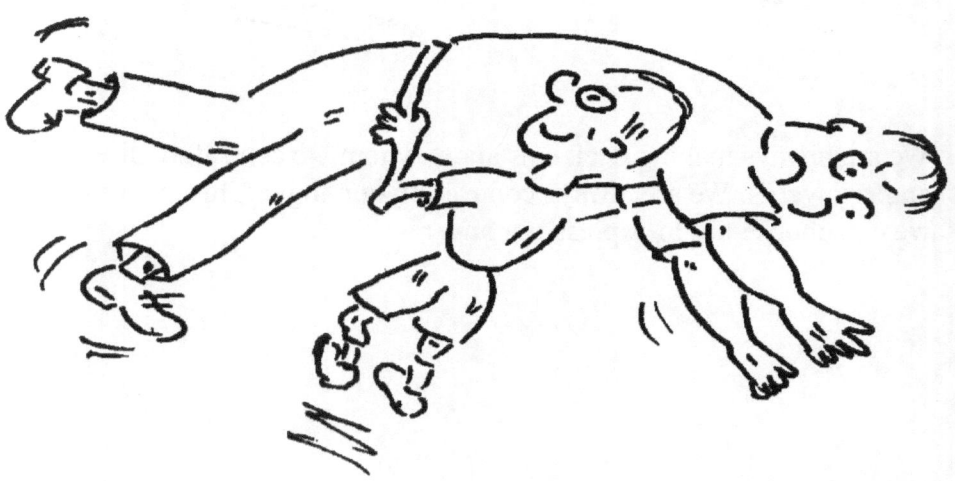

Fear

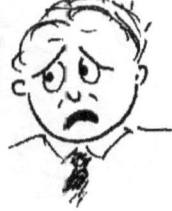

Shame

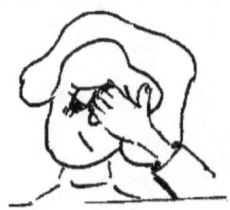

Guilt

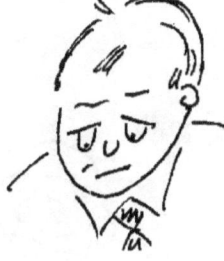

are our alternatives to anger.

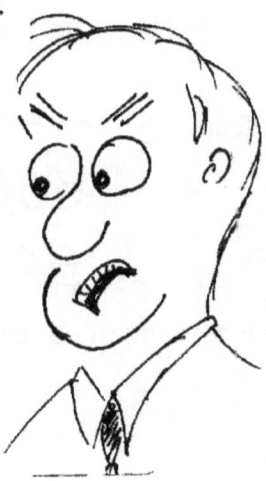

They offer us the opportunity to deal with the
underlying problem, instead of becoming angry.

Our ability to control our anger,
by examining our underlying

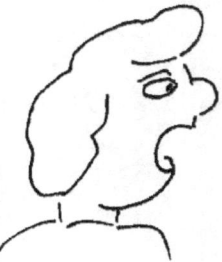

shame

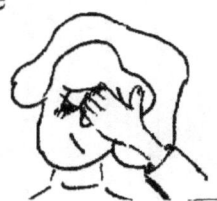

guilt

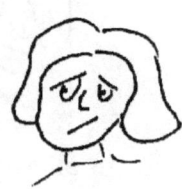

or fear

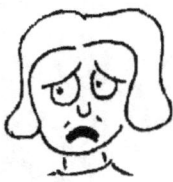

is a measure of our psychological maturity.

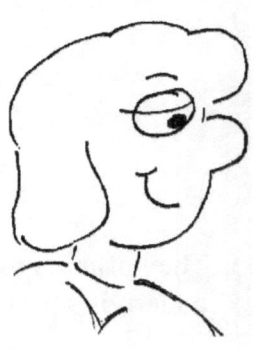

We become angry when we cannot deal with the issues that threaten us, or about which we feel guilty or ashamed.

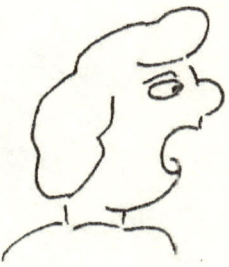

To abort our anger, we must admit that we are feeling:

threatened

ashamed

or guilty

and deal with the issues.

Anger creates anger. Expressing anger [catharsis] never solves an anger problem for those who have issues from the past.

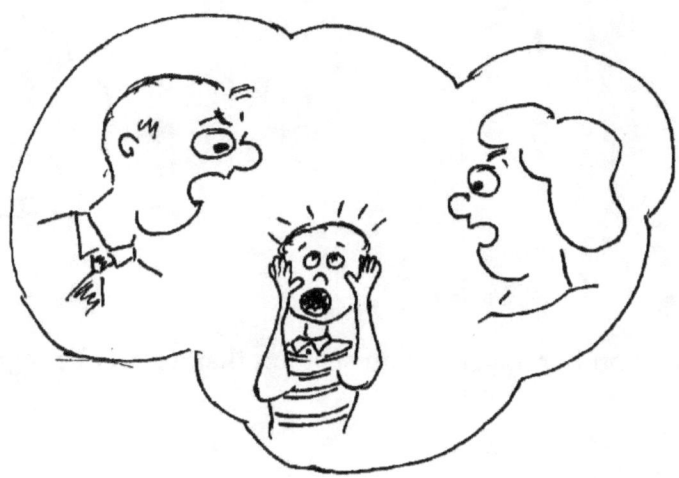

Catharsis may cause a degree of exhaustion that brings temporary relief.

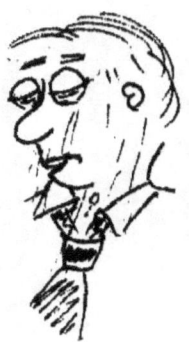

However, such behaviour simply emphasizes the:

Fear

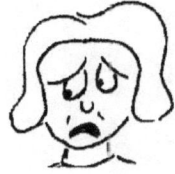

Guilt

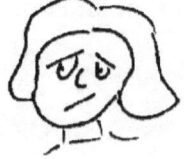

and Shame

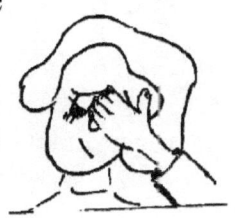

that we have from our past.

There are three types of anger :

Regular anger with shouting and physical violence.

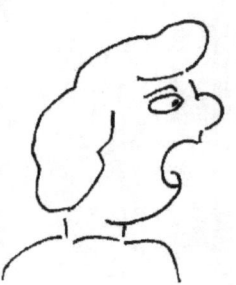

Hidden anger with obstructive behaviour, verbal and emotional abuse.

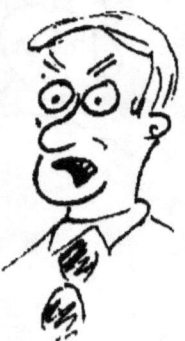

And anger directed inwards causing depression.

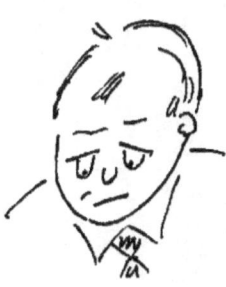

Suicide is the most violent expression of anger directed inwards,

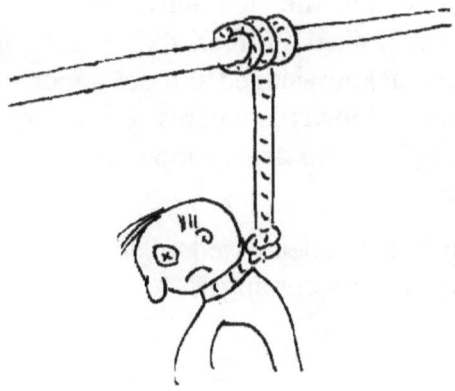

as murder is the most violent expression of anger directed outwards.

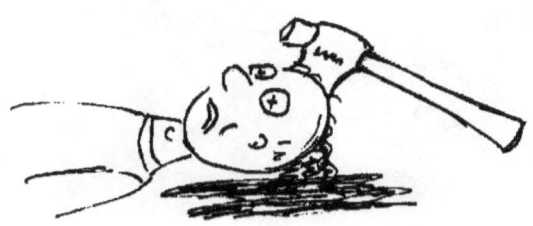

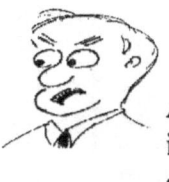

Anger can be directed outwards or inwards. When our fear, shame and guilt are not acknowledged and our anger is directed inwards, depression occurs, although not all depression comes from anger.

Some of us may become depressed when we are unable to express our anger.

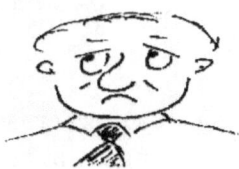

When we are unable to acknowledge,

fear

shame

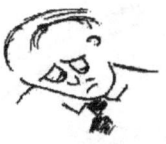

or guilt.

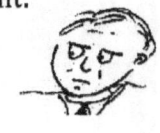

Some of us become depressed; we harm ourselves rather than harm others.

In order to be relieved of our depression

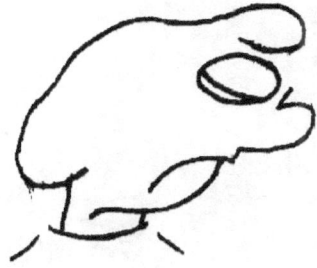

we need help to expose our anger and deal with our:

fear

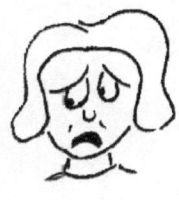

guilt

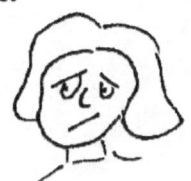

or shame

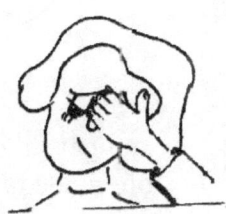

Hidden anger has to be exposed and acknowledged. Only then can we admit our:

Shame

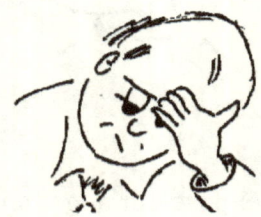

Guilt

or Fear

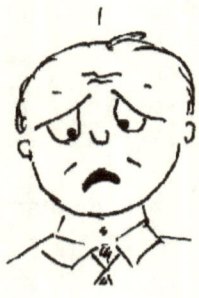

and get rid of our anger. Those who are hiding anger often need help to expose it.

Passive resistance and silence are often the only expression of anger in a relationship.

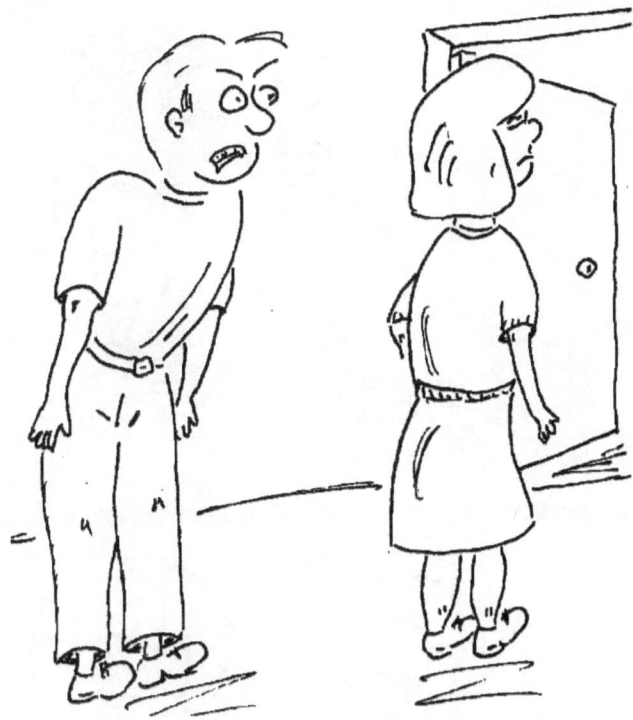

They are used by the angry person who is unable to confront another person.

A sense of injustice is one of the greatest psychological threats.

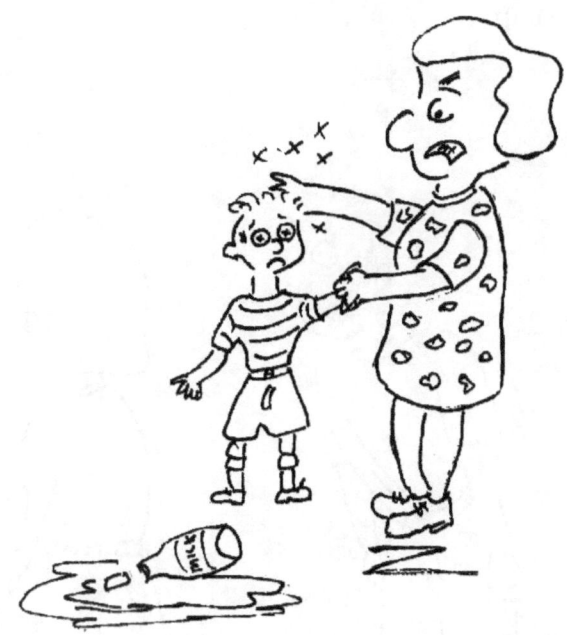

It may prevail over many years and across great distances.

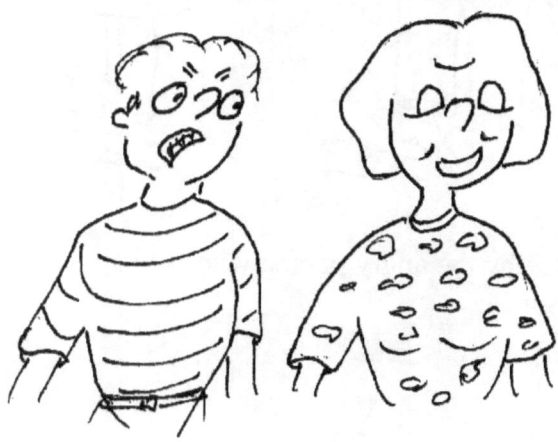

Extreme anger and violence

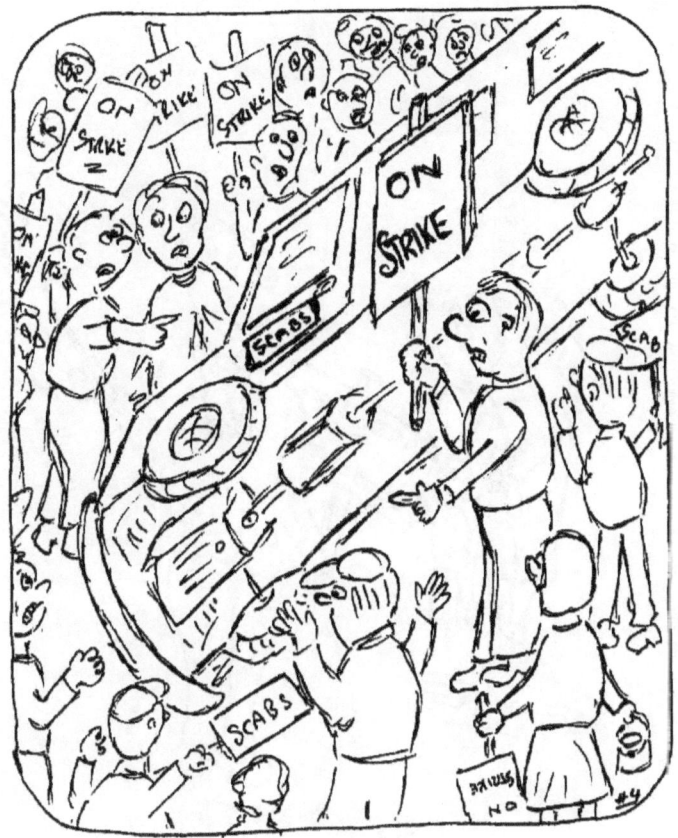

may result from a sense of injustice.

The feeling of injustice occurs...

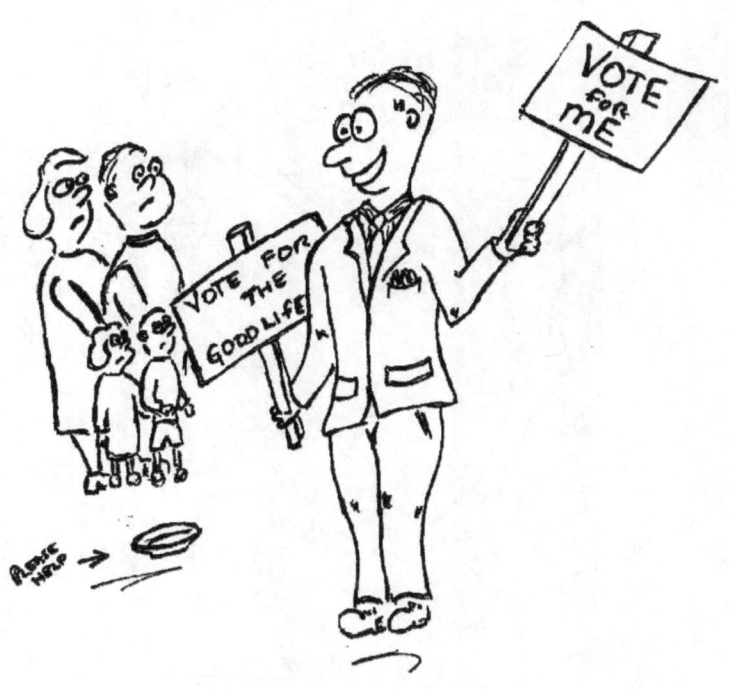

when our expectations are not met.

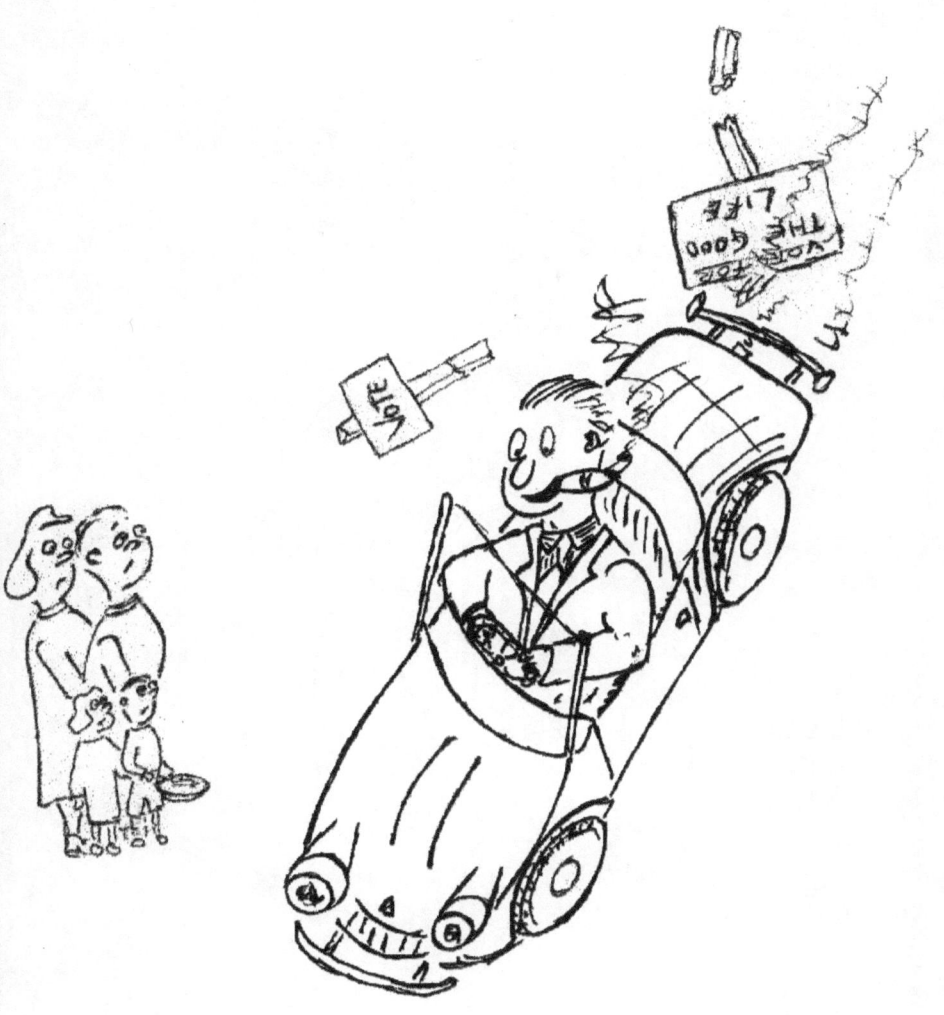

The more we expect the more resentful we get when our expectations are not met.

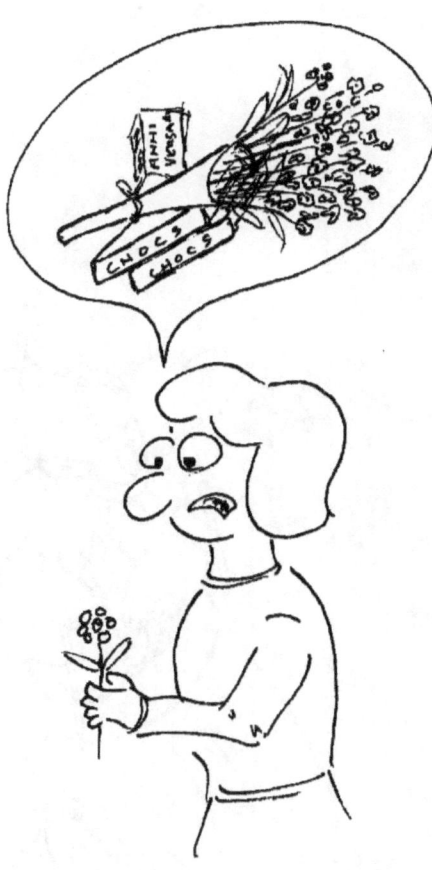

We may get angry when promises made to us are broken.

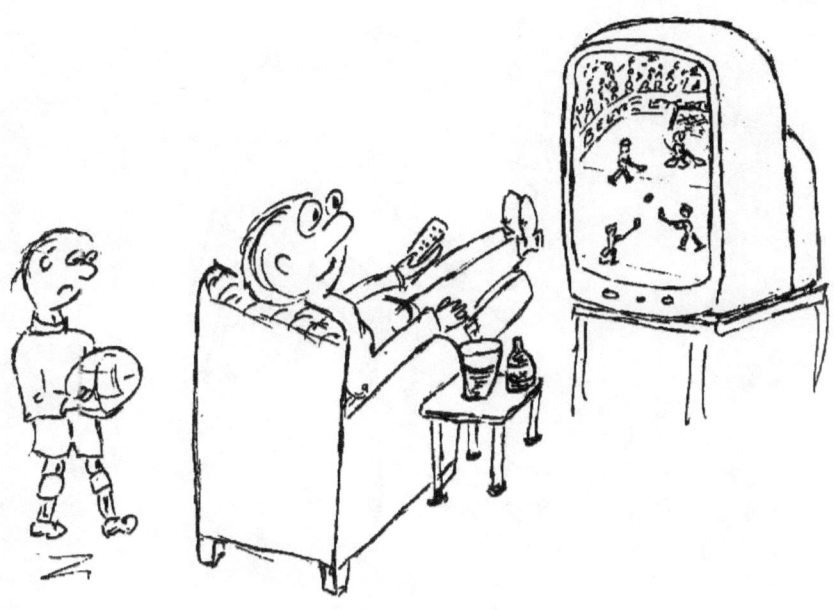

Poor self-esteem can be a cause of ongoing anger.

The insecure person easily feels threatened and may have an anger problem. In such cases the poor self-esteem may need to be treated, in order to get rid of the anger problem.

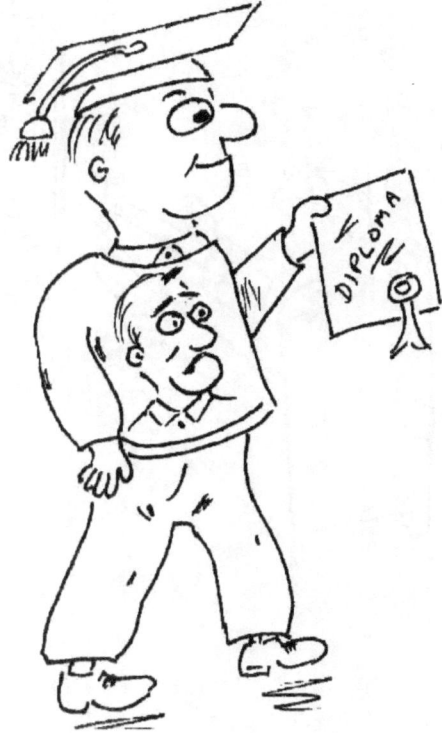

Level of achievement does not determine whether or not a person is insecure and angry.

Some people may not develop the ability to feel shame and guilt.

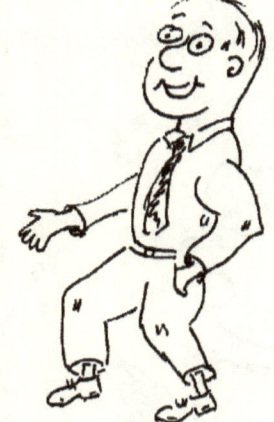

They leave a trail of violence and destruction behind them.

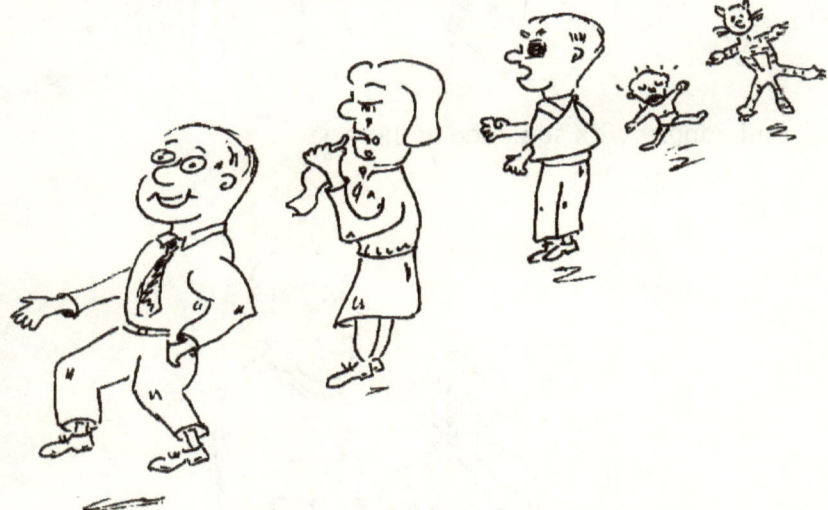

These unfortunate people are called psychopaths.

The person to whom our anger is directed may not be the cause of our anger.
We may direct our anger at someone in the present when we

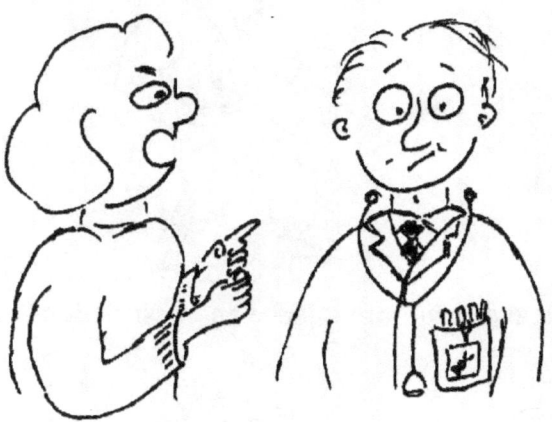

really angry with someone in the past.

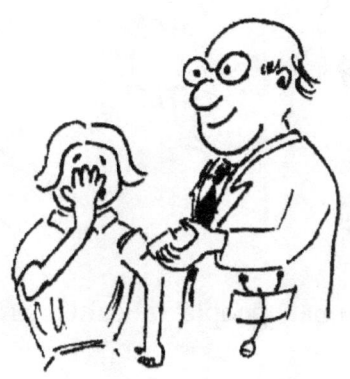

Something about the innocent person in the present reminds our subconscious of a time in the past when we felt:

Fear

Shame

or Guilt

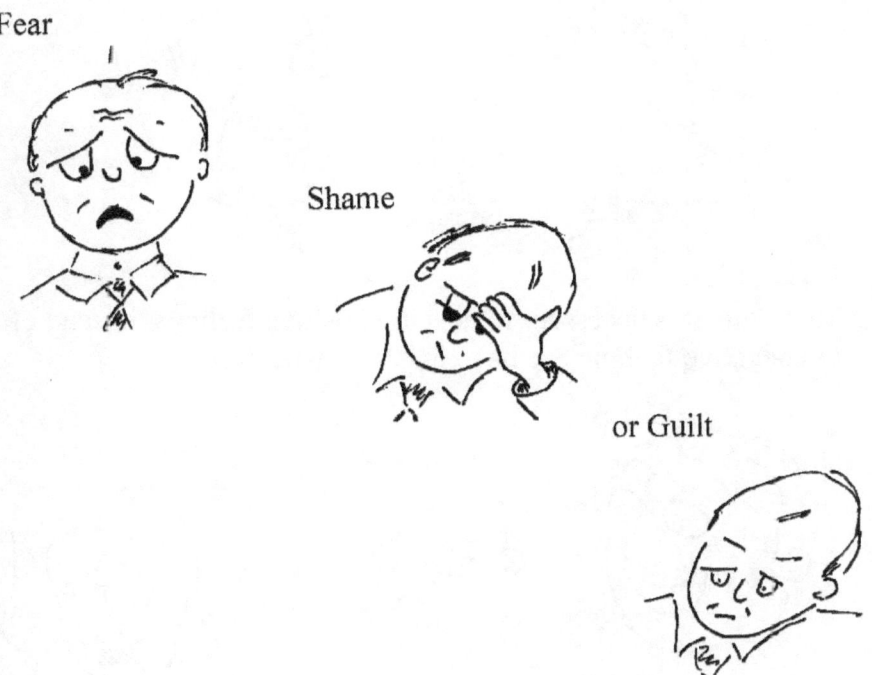

In such situations the present degree of anger is usually out of all proportion to the apparent cause. The degree of anger cannot be understood in terms of the present issue. Our hidden conflicts of the past are unknowingly applied to the present. This is called 'Transference'.

The only way to get rid of our anger from the past is to come to terms with past events.

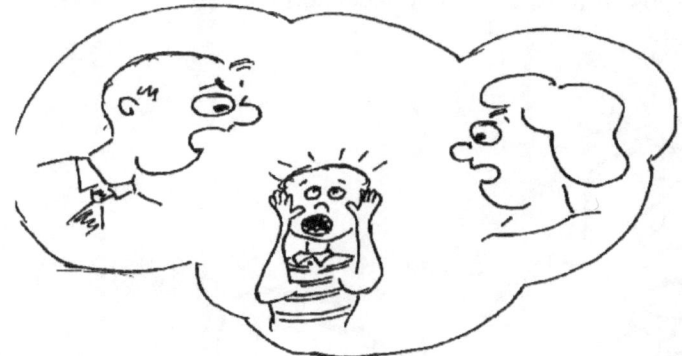

To do this it is necessary to develop positive feelings, instead of the negative feelings we have for those who hurt us.

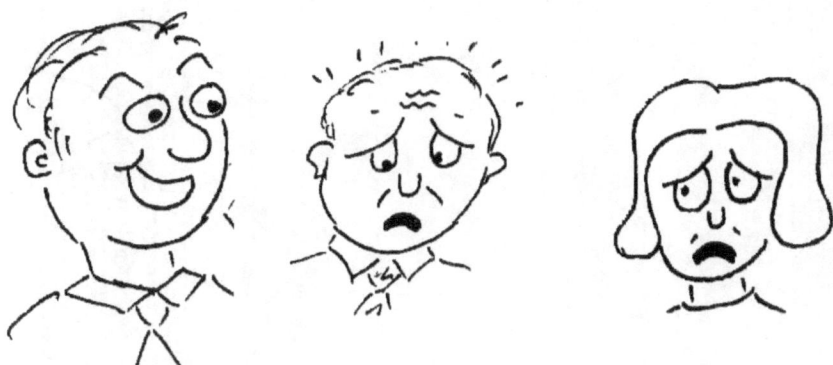

Those who have hurt us were hurt themselves when they were children. By understanding the mechanism of anger it is often possible to find reasons to feel sorry for those who have hurt us.

Eventually, peace of mind may come by forgiving them. It is not necessary to confront those who have hurt us in order to resolve our anger, although meeting and talking to them can lead to understanding, sometimes.

The mechanism of anger.

To understand anger we need to have some knowledge of the
Autonomic Nervous Sytem, [A.N.S.]

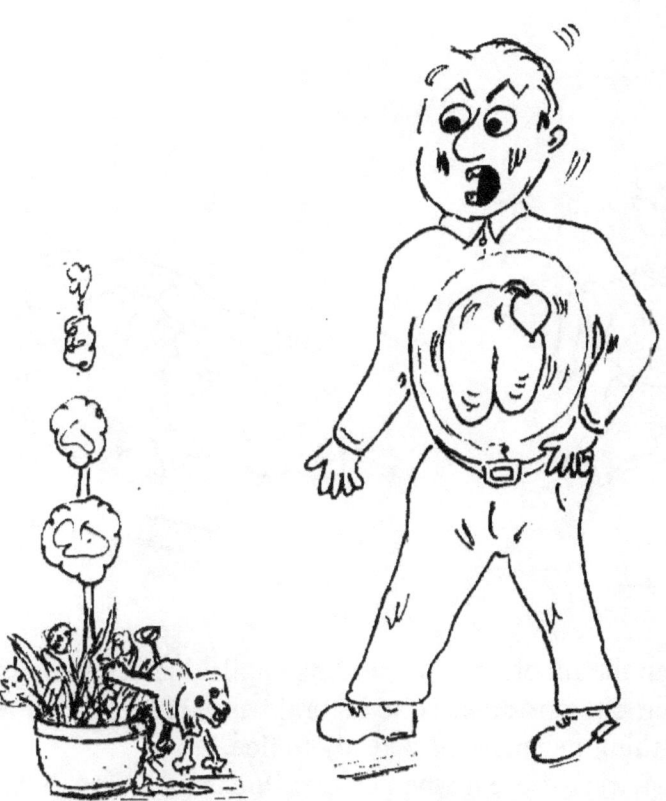

The A.N.S. governs those parts of the body that we are
not normally aware of e.g.- heart rate, blood pressure,
contraction of the pupils.

We cannot live without A.N.S.

The Autonomic Nervous System is influenced by our higher brain centers, but it is also present in all creatures that do not have such centers.

The A.N.S. is the primitive nervous system that allows all creatures to respond to danger.

It allows us to turn and flee, stand and fight, or hide and freeze.

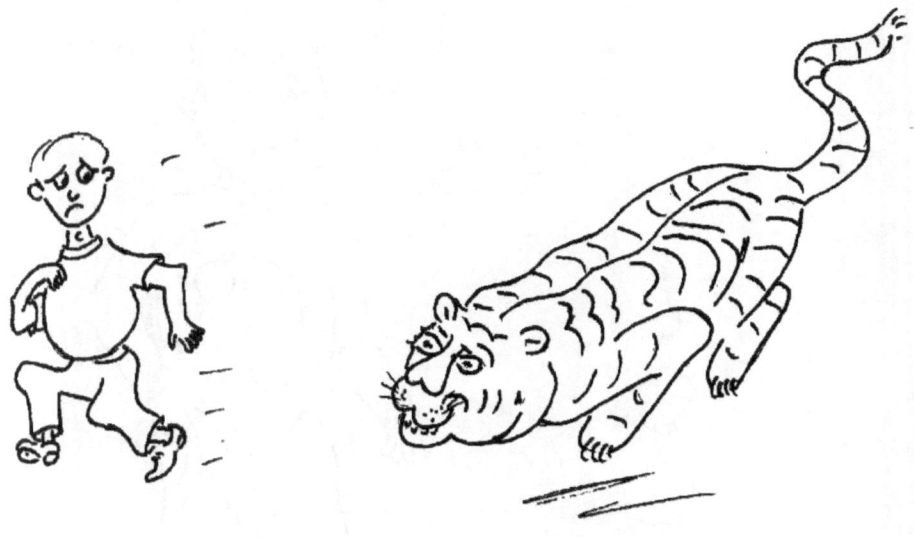

When the rabbit sees the fox, its pupils dilate, its heart beats faster, blood is diverted to its brain and limbs and its rate of breathing increases. It is ready to flee.

We are no different when danger threatens. Our A.N.S. activates, preparing us to flee or stand and fight. It is active when we feel anxious or angry.

Continuous peak activity of the A.N.S. is exhausting and cannot be maintained.

Anger directed outwards extends from simple frustration to rage,

Frustration

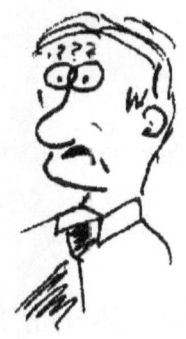

Anger

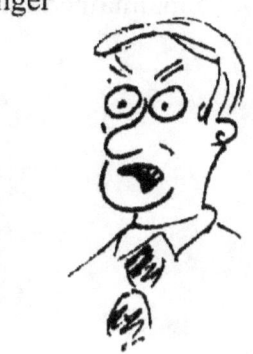

Rage

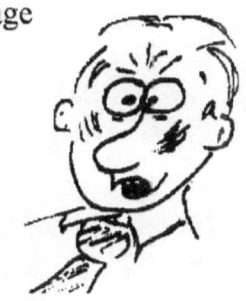

with a corresponding increase in autonomic nervous activity.

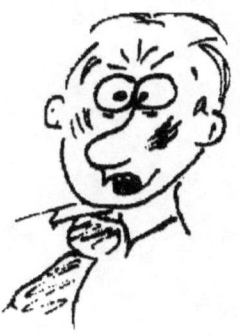

Rage, with peak activity of the autonomic nervous system, is exhausting and cannot be maintained for any great length of time.

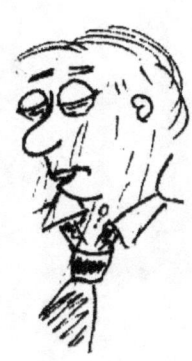

Many things stimulate the Autonomic Nervous Sytem
e.g.- exposure to the anger of others,

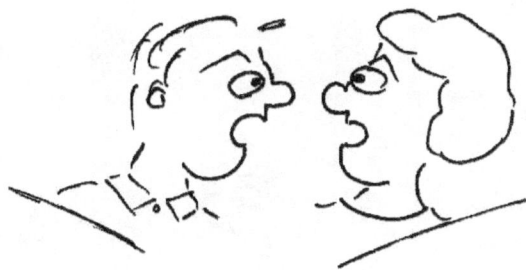

loud noise, observing violence, anticipation of confrontation.
If our A.N.S. activity is already elevated further stimulation
will increase its activity.

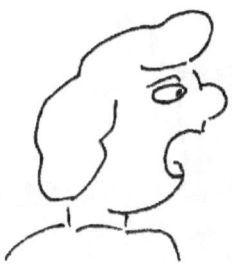

There is an accumulative effect.

An event that would not normally provoke anger may do so if
A.N.S. activity is already increased.

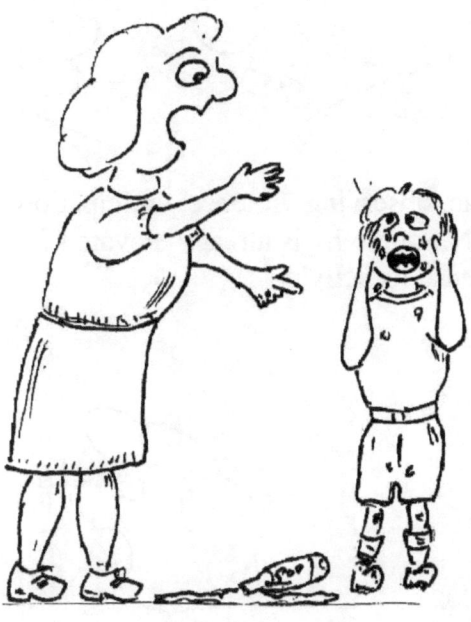

A low level of autonomic nervous activity, associated with   simmering anger, can be maintained over many years.

It is a burden.

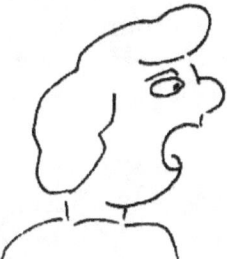

It means that the:

Fear

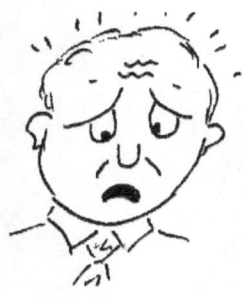

Guilt

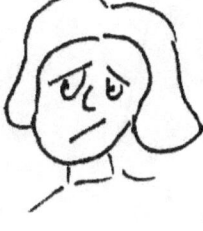

Shame

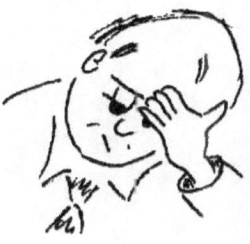

from the past have not been acknowledged, and dealt with.

We can reduce the level of our anger, with relaxation exercises that reverse the activity of our Autonomic Nervous System.

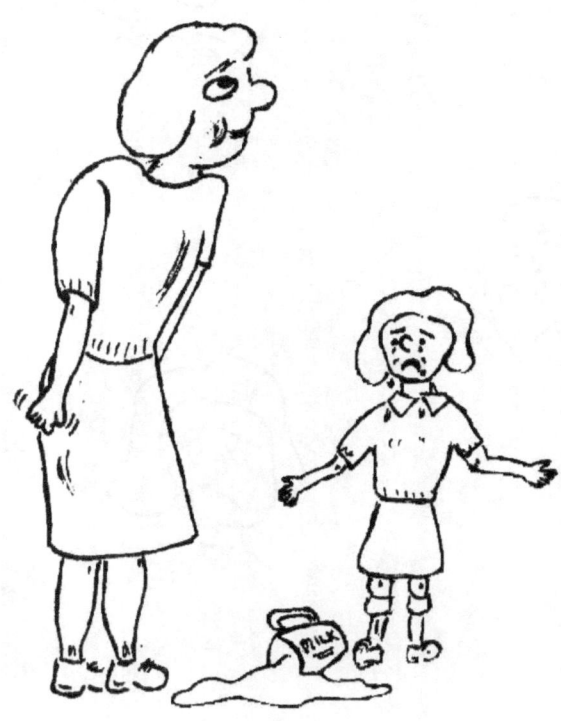

However, to get rid of our anger we need to acknowledge our shame, guilt or fear.

Our Autonomic Nervous System is also activated for positive reasons.
Positive stress is activity of the A.N.S. with positive emotions. It is always healthy.

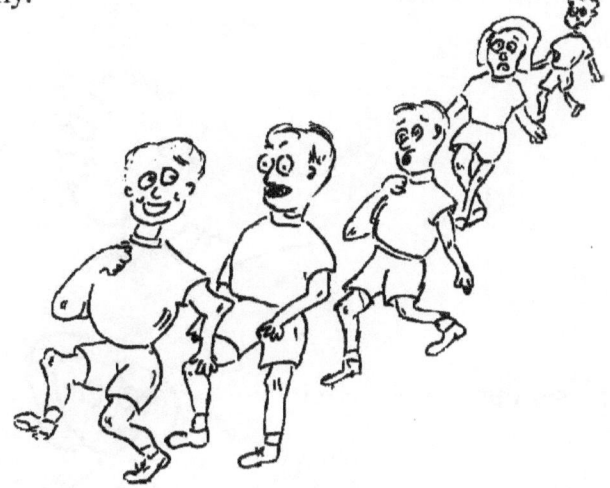

Negative stress is activity of the A.N.S. with negative emotions. It is unhealthy when continuous.

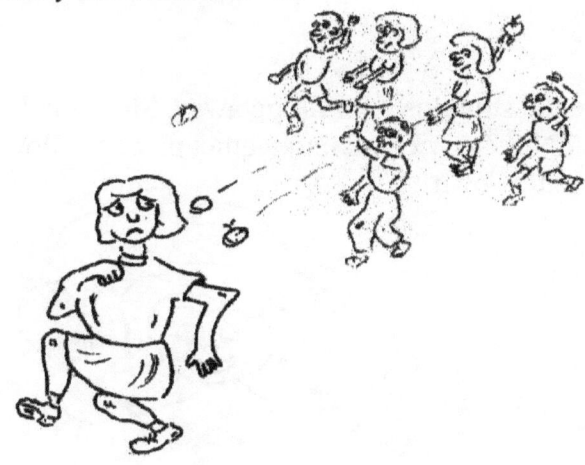

The relationship of anger to the Autonomic Nervous System explains some of the traditional ways we deal with anger.

When anger in others

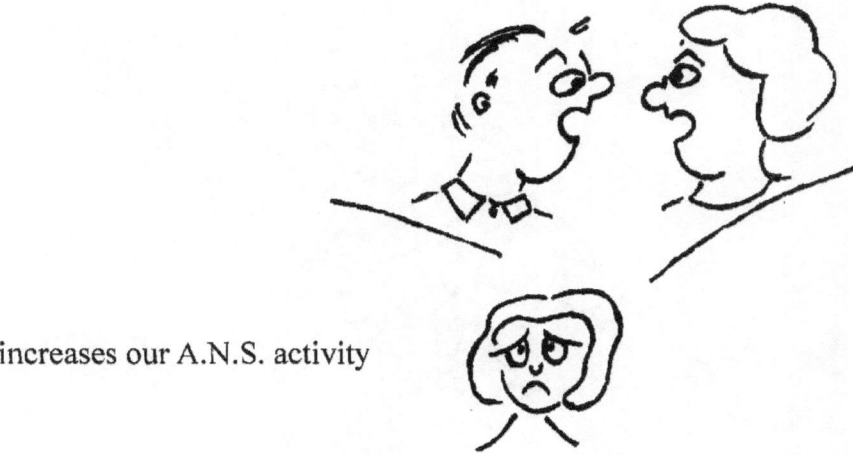

increases our A.N.S. activity

we remove the stimulus by walking away. Since loud noise increases A.N.S. activity we find a quiet place to allow our A.N.S. to settle down.

Slow, deep breaths help reduce the level of Autonomic Nervous System activity. We are the only creature that can deliberately slow the rate of breathing.
By doing so we are actually reversing the activity of the A.N.S.

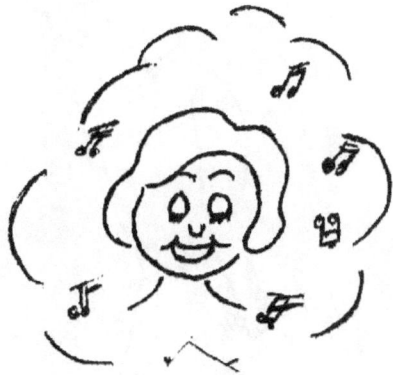

Evolution has provided us, through our higher brain centers, a means to directly influence A.N.S. activity and our anger.

These traditional ways of controlling our anger are important.

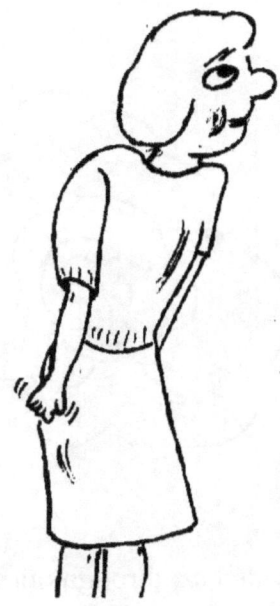

However, they are only dealing with the symptom not the condition.

Anger comes from the emotions of:

Fear

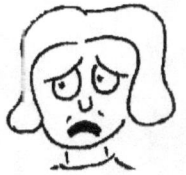

Guilt

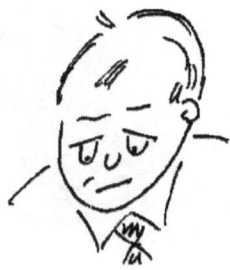

Shame

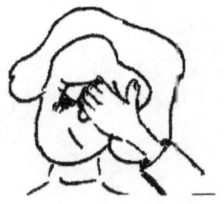

The Autonomic Nervous System can become conditioned to respond to a situation.
The situation may be a major traumatic event as in the Post Traumatic Stress Syndrome

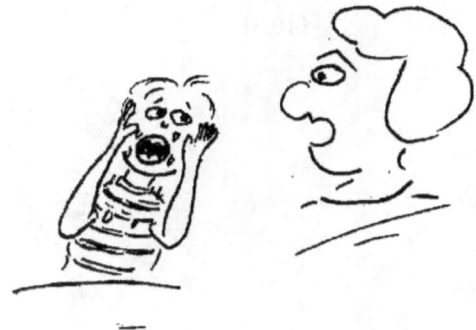

or repeated events during childhood and adolesence.

Continuous loud and aggressive verbal abuse may cause elevation of A.N.S. when we are exposed to such behaviour as adults.

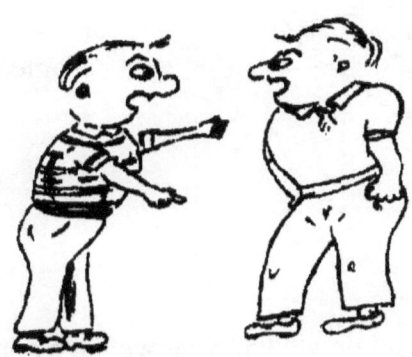

Adults with an anger problem often have a family history of such behaviour.

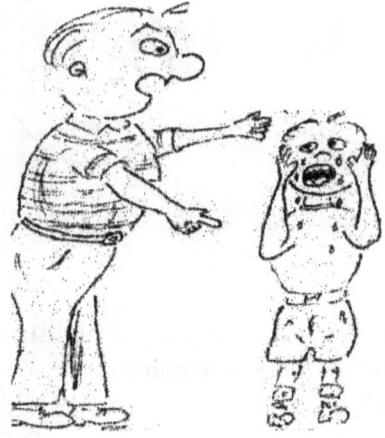

If we are feeling:

guilty

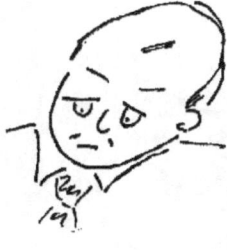

or
ashamed

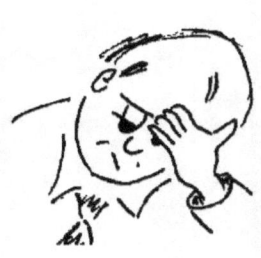

we need to acknowledge what we have done wrong and apologize to the person we have hurt.

If we feel threatened

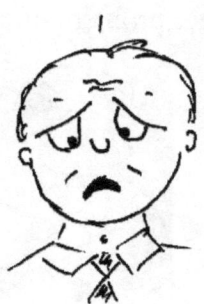

we need to express and share our feelings in a way that is not threatening to the person we are angry with.

The emotional origins and physiology of anger are the same for both men and women.

Traditionally, in western society, women have not occupied positions of power in public life. Anger and violence in public, by women, has therefore been far less than that expressed and committed by men.

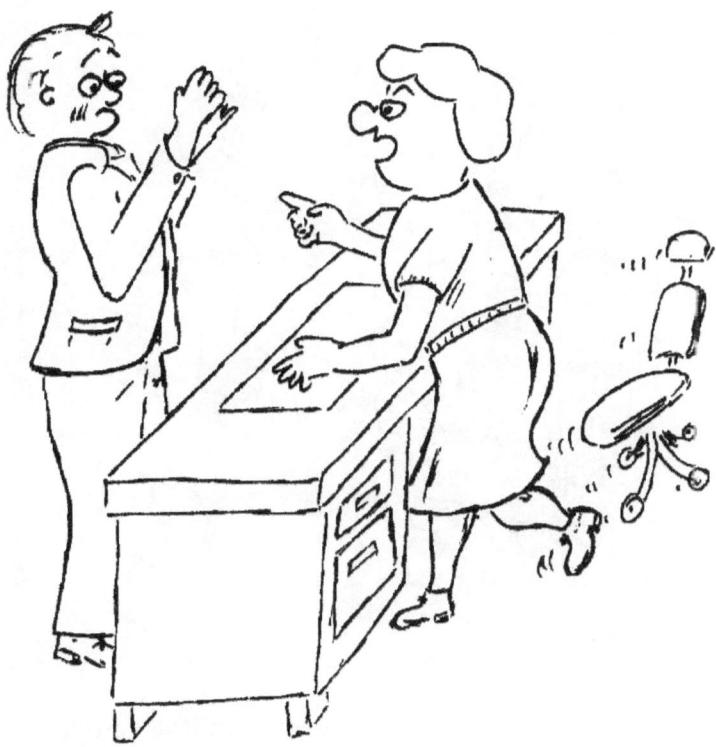

As women assume positions of authority and power in society, we can expect them to express more anger and commit more violence, in the manner traditionally attributed to men.

CONTROLLING OUR ANGER

We cannot control our anger when we are under the influence of alcohol.

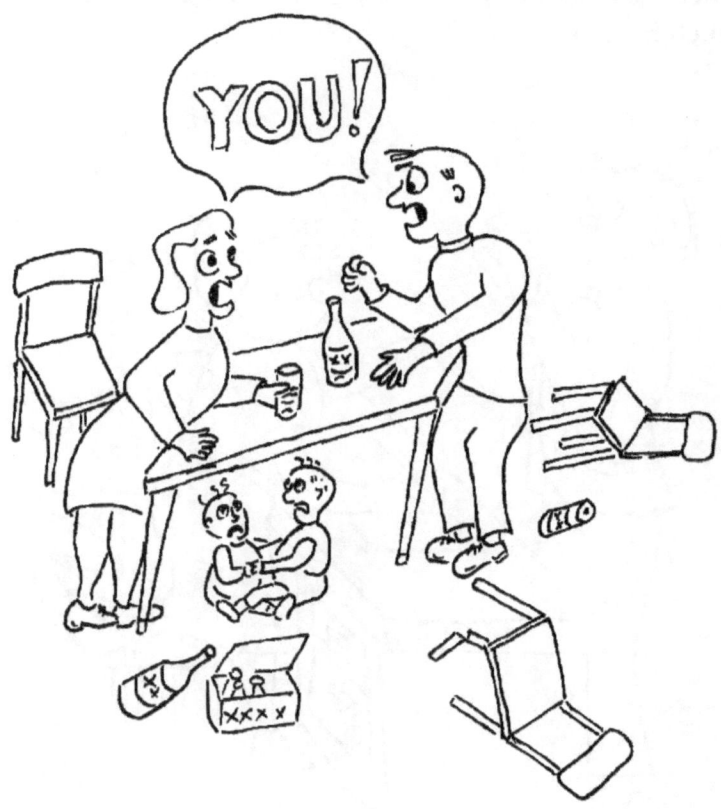

If alcohol is an issue it needs to be dealt with if we are to control our anger.

Understand the emotional origins of anger, as previously outlined.

When we feel angry, we should ask ourselves " Why am I feeling angry? Am I feeling threatened, ashamed or guilty?"

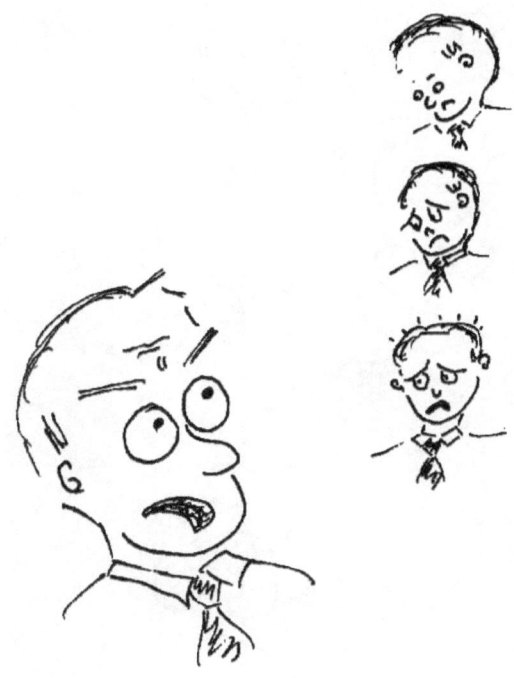

It may be all three emotions, although they will not be felt simultaneously.

Having established which emotion[s] is underlying the anger, ask "Why am I feeling threatened, ashamed or guilty?"

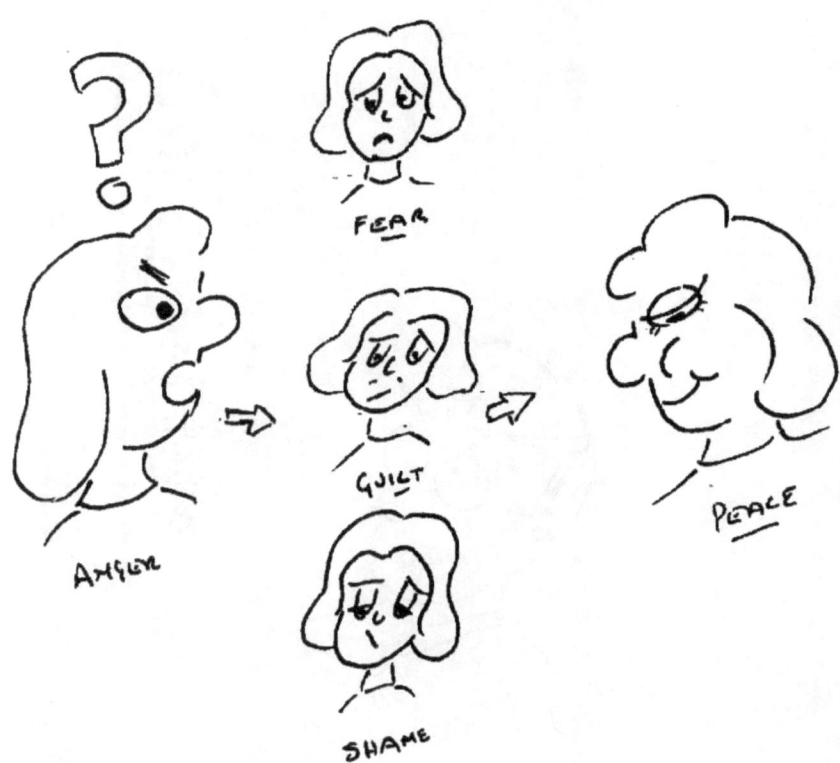

Then deal with the issues.

Some very insecure people feel guilty or ashamed all the time about issues that they are not responsible for.

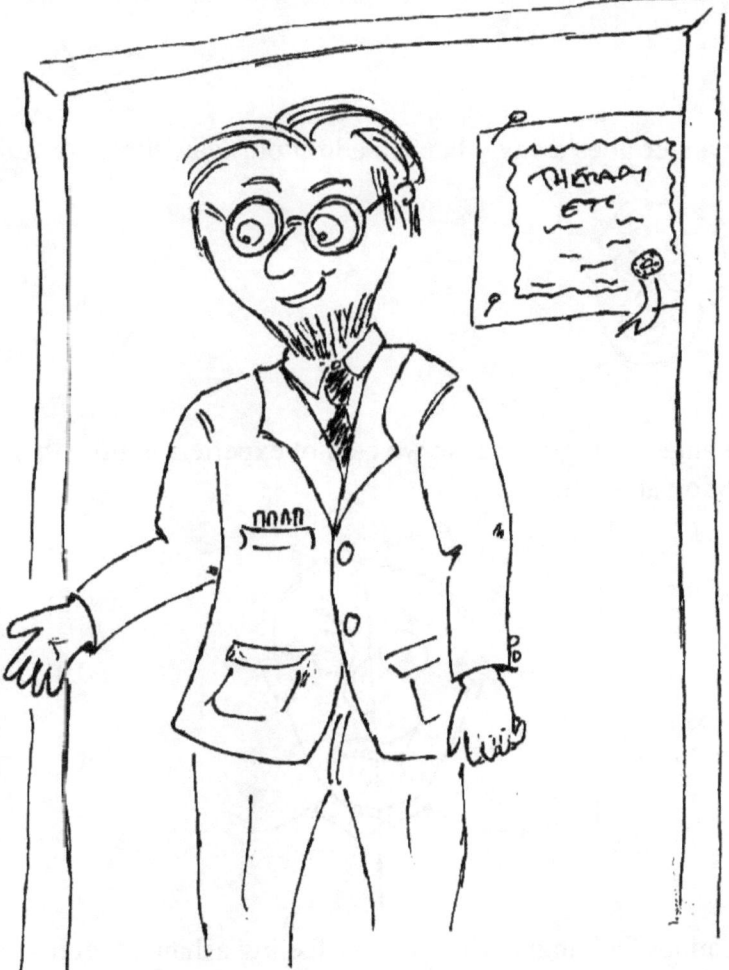

They need help to rid themselves of their burden of fear, shame or guilt.

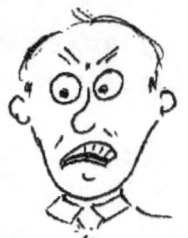

Our anger goes away when we admit our fear, shame or guilt.

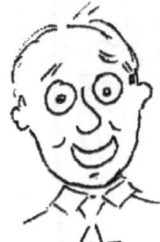

The anger will go because we cannot experience more than one emotion at a time.

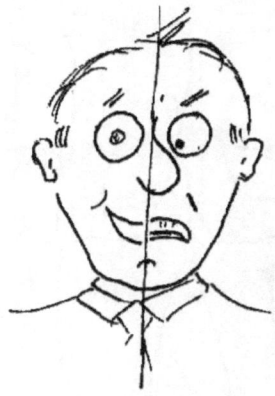

We cannot feel angry while we are feeling ashamed, guilty or frightened.
It is not easy to admit our shame, guilt or fear.
We may need help.
The more insecure we are in ourselves the more difficult it is.

We need to recognize when we are continually angry, often over trivial events.

Ask, "Why am I continually feeling threatened, ashamed or guilty?" and acknowledge and deal with the issue, with help if necessary.

We must ask ourselves

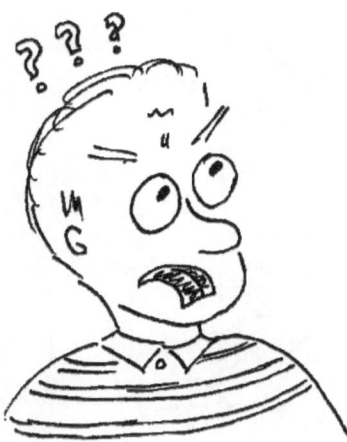

what is it that is bothering us and whether it is something from our past.

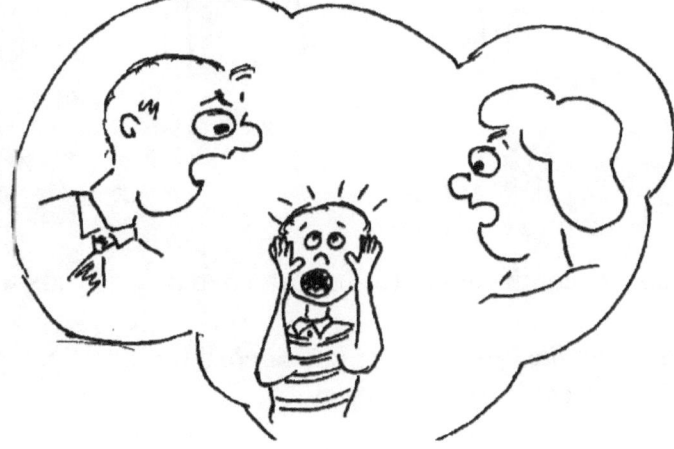

Dealing with the issue is often difficult and painful, which is why we become angry in the first place.
We may need help to face the underlying emotions of fear, guilt or shame.

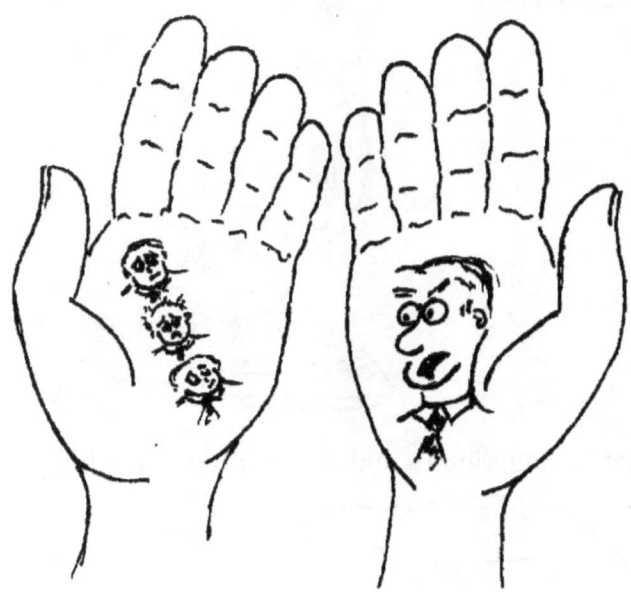

It is not easy to admit we are feeling ashamed or guilty about something.
It is often difficult to admit we are threatened by something and then deal with the threat in a positive way.

When anger has been present since childhood,

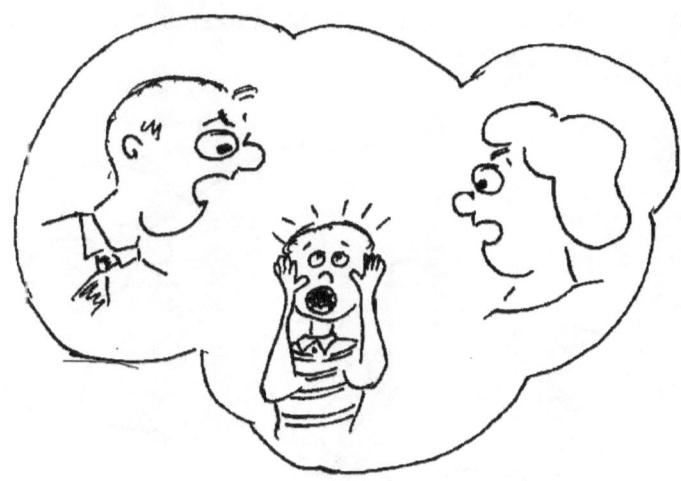

it is usually necessary to have professional
help in dealing with
       Fear
           Guilt
               Shame
that originates from childhood events.
Under no circumstances should this result in
laying blame on those who have hurt us in the
past.

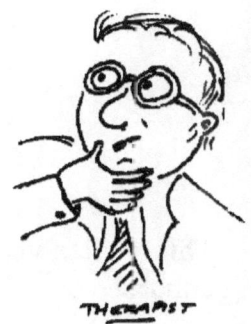

THERAPIST

If we feel sorry for those who have hurt us our
anger will go away

Blaming others only feeds our anger. Certainly, the role others have played in causing fear, shame or guilt needs to be acknowledged.
However, it needs to be acknowledged in such a way as not to lay blame or promote anger.

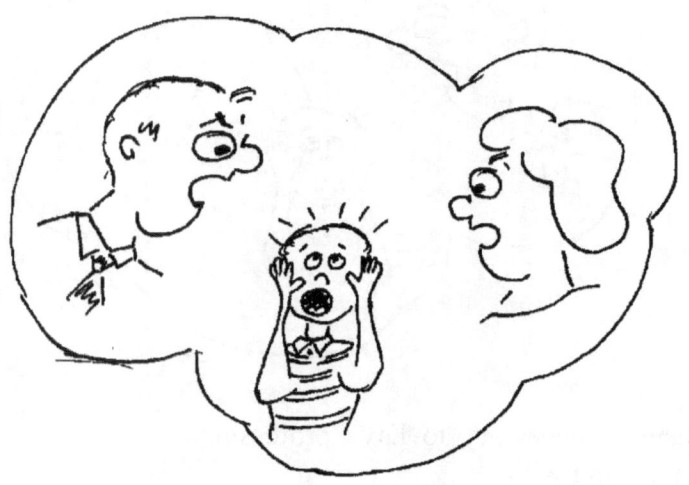

This is often very difficult, but there is no alternative if we wish to unburden ourselves of our anger.

Remember transference from page 35
When another person's anger is great and the cause trivial, we may not be the true cause of their anger.

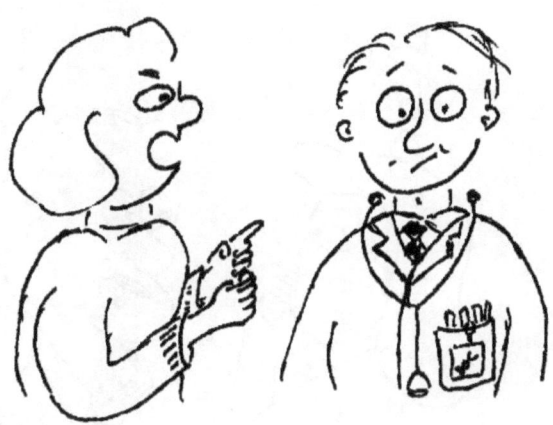

In such cases they are really angry with someone else from their past, recent or distant, although they are unaware of the fact.

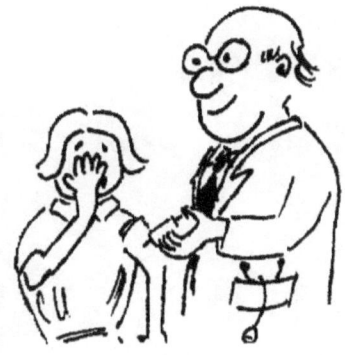

If someone is angry with us, ask "why is this person angry? Are they feeling threatened, guilty, or ashamed?"

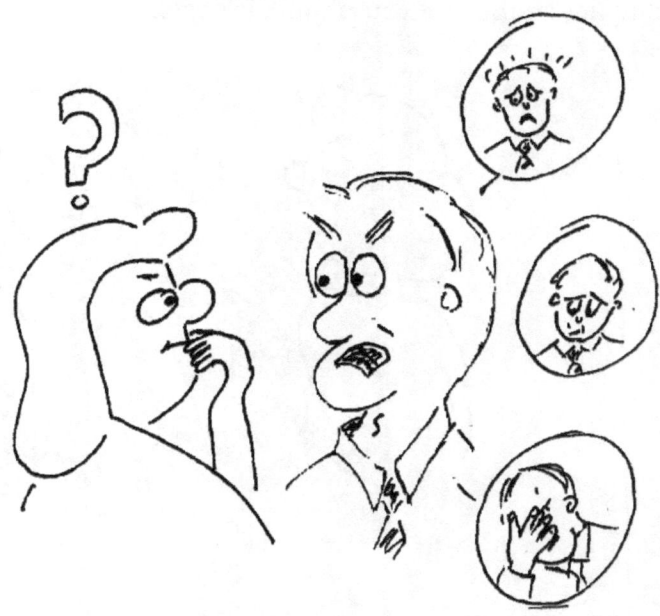

In this way we may understand the person who is confronting us.

We must learn to reduce exposure to Autonomic Nervous System stimulation.

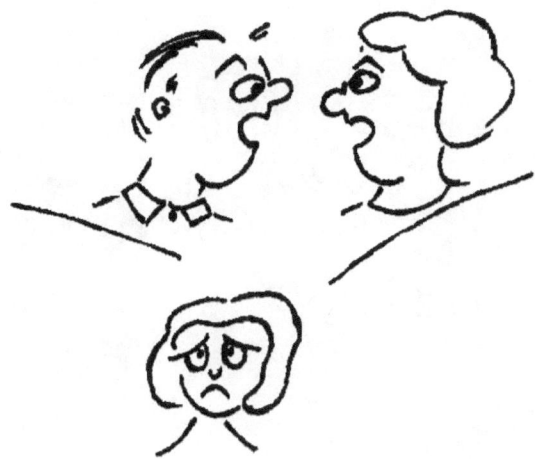

Apply all the traditional methods such as finding a quiet place, taking deep breaths and other relaxing exercises.

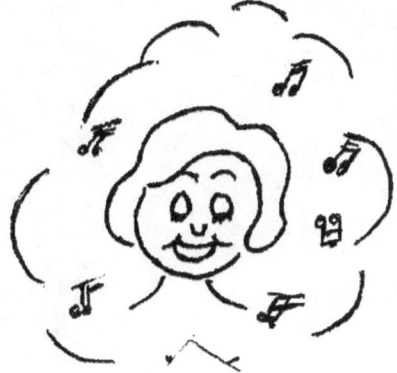

Continuous feeling of inadequacy and insecurity needs to be addressed if the problem of ongoing anger is to be resolved

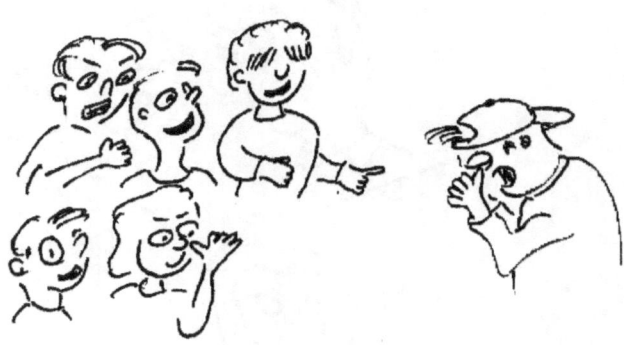

and tragedy avoided.

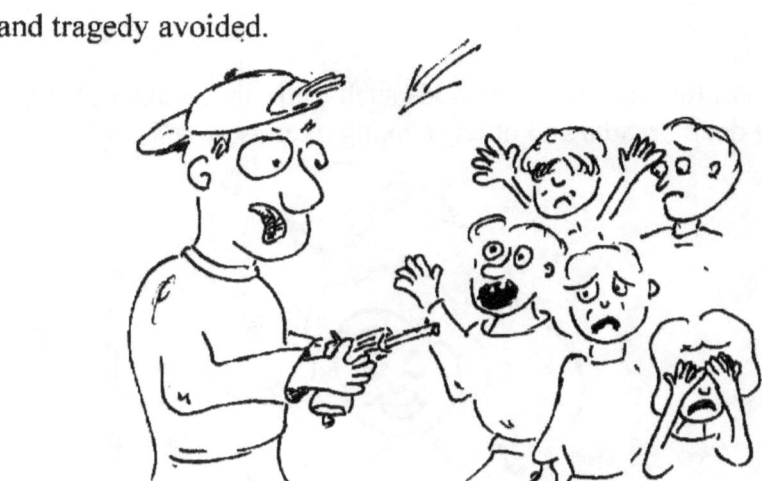

HOW TO TALK WHEN THE OTHER PERSON IS ANGRY

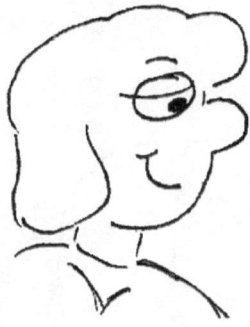 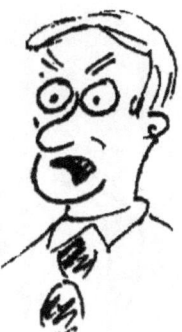

In a friendly conversation, if we use "I" all the time, we create the impression that we think too much of ourselves. This irritates the person we are talking to.

The art of conversation is to use "you". i.e. - "How are you?" "What do you think of this?"

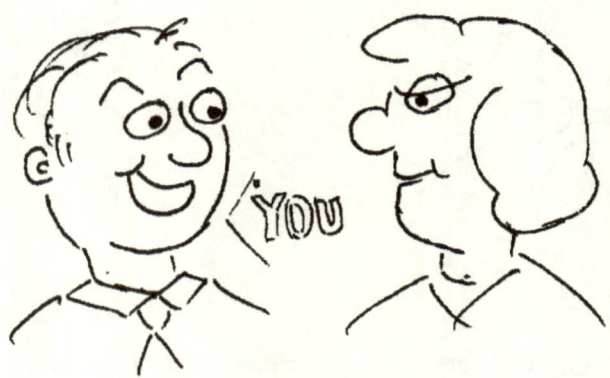

Then listen to the answer.

Normally we use "you" all the time in an argument. This is bad.

When we say "you" in an argument, we push the other person away from us and cause them to feel threatened.

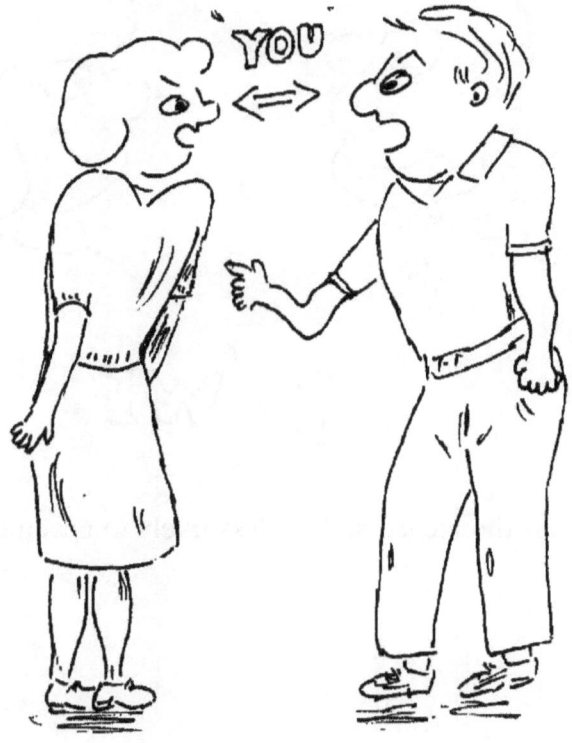

The person who feels threatened is likely to get angry. The argument increases.

When we use I [and we] in an argument we draw the other person to us.

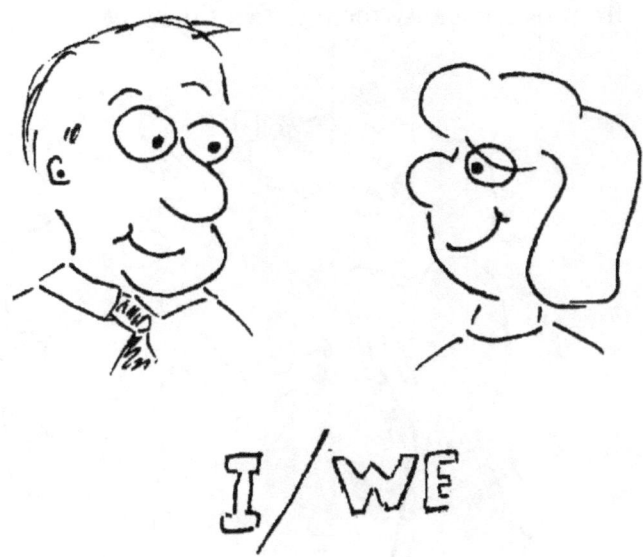

They feel less threatened and are less likely to become angry.

Normally in an argument we tell the other person what we think.

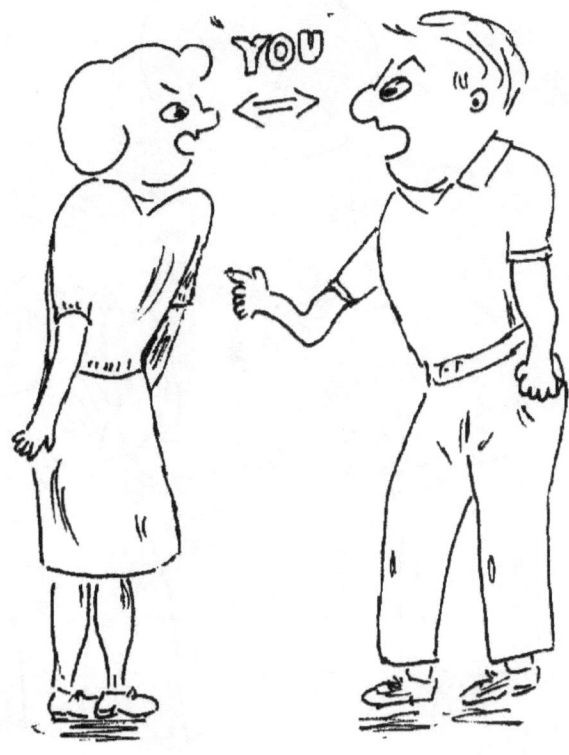

It is easy to be angry with someone who tells you what they think about you.

e.g.-"I think you are mean for saying that to me."

In an argument we must tell the other person what we are feeling, not what we are thinking.

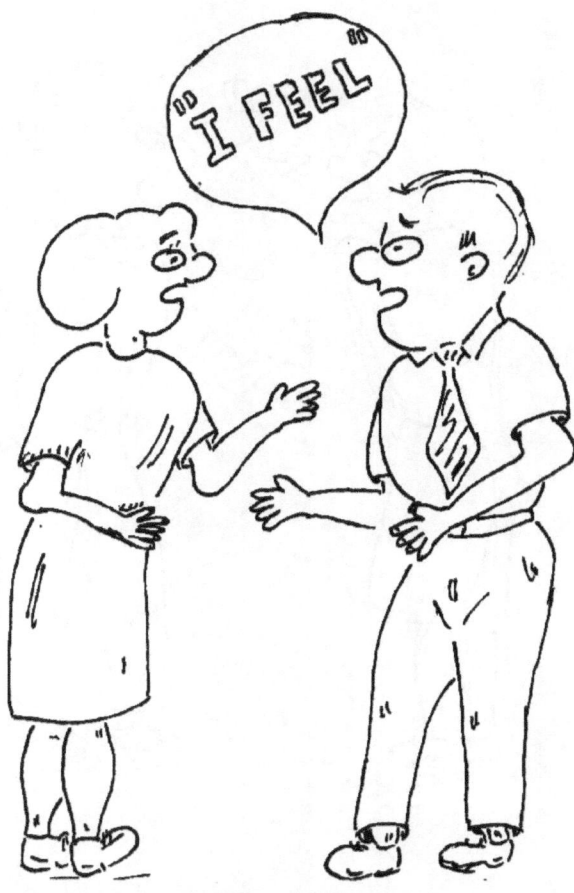

It is difficult to be angry with someone who is sharing with us how they feel inside.

e.g.-"It hurts me when I am spoken to like this."

So, in a confrontational situation-

Use "I" and "We"

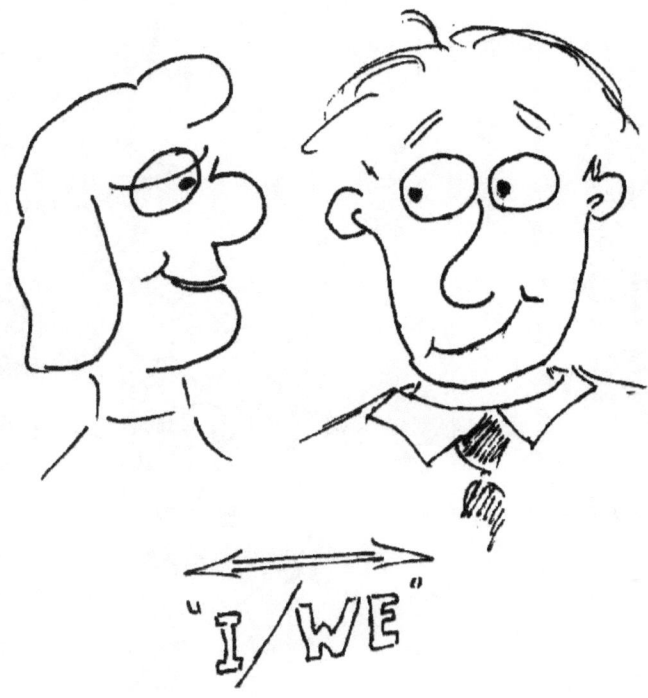

and let the other person know what you are feeling.

CHANGING OUR THOUGHTS AND EMOTIONS

We can only think one thought at a time.
We can only feel one emotion at a time.

We cannot have a positive and negative thought at the same time.

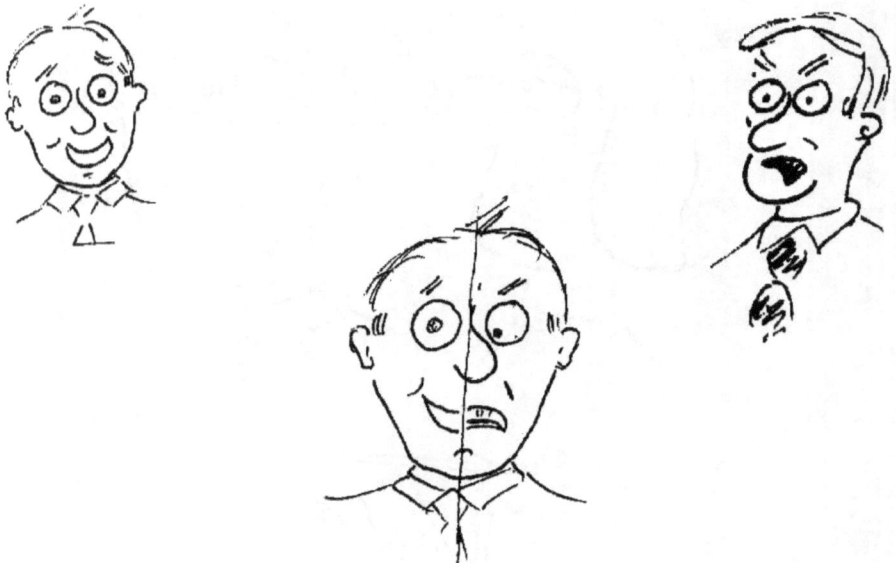

We cannot feel a positive and a negative emotion at the same time.

Thoughts influence emotions and emotions influence thoughts.

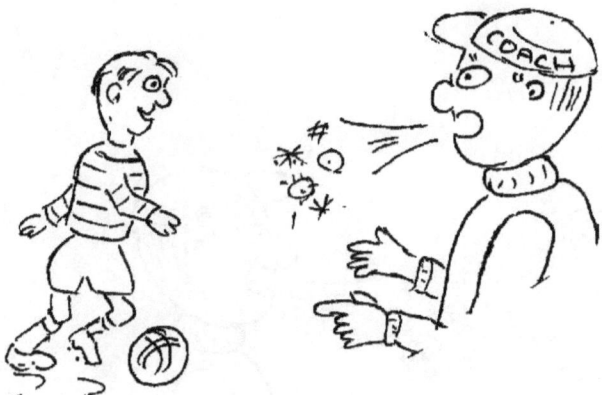

For the sad and the lonely depressed person, most thoughts are negative.

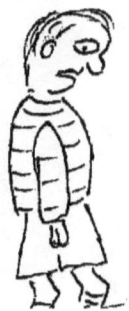

Those who think they are stupid and inferior will feel sad and lonely.

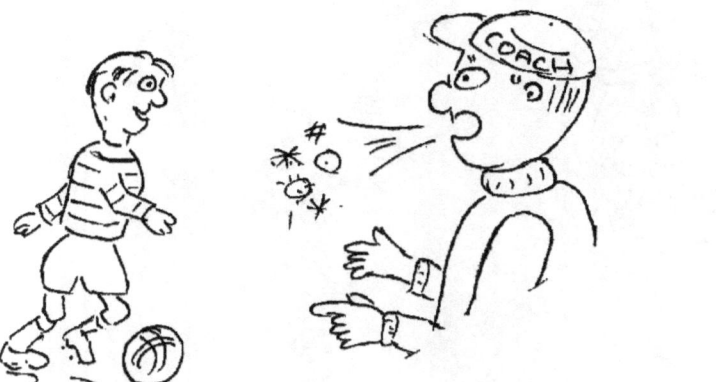

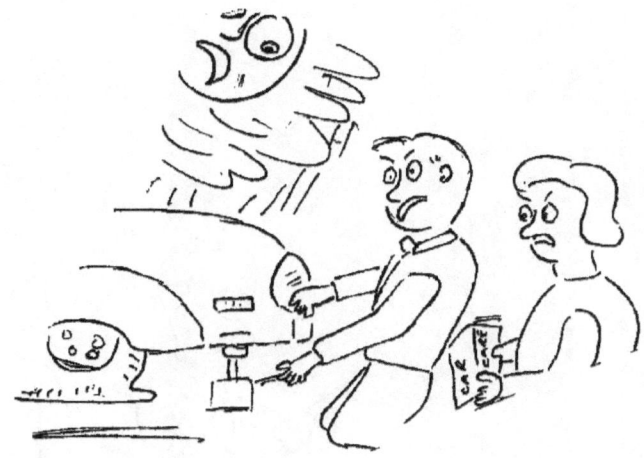

By thinking a positive thought we are able to develop other positive thoughts and also develop positive emotions.

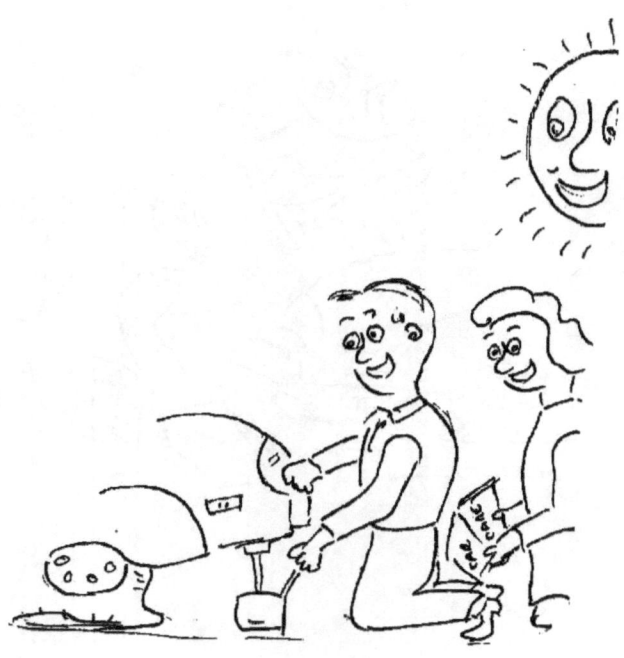

By feeling a positive emotion we can develop positive thoughts.

When we are angry we are feeling the negative emotions of shame, guilt or fear,

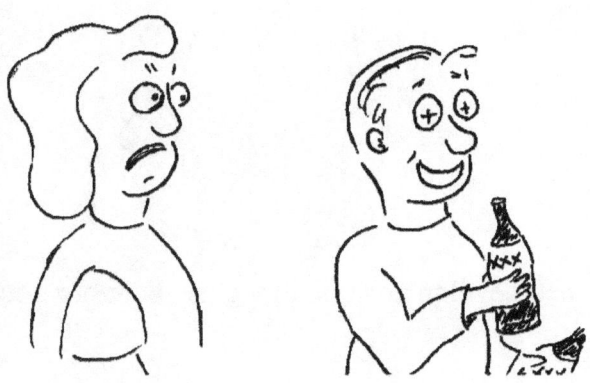

while we are also thinking hostile, negative thoughts.

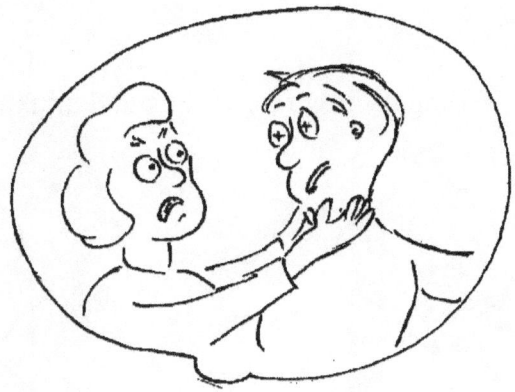

To be relieved of our anger we need to replace the negative emotions of shame, guilt or fear with a positive emotion.

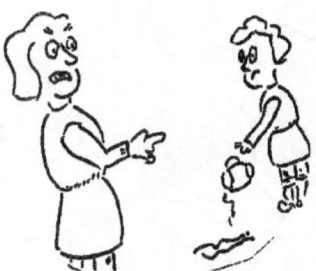

We can then develop positive thoughts about our situation.

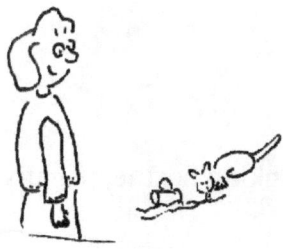

We cannot be angry if we are feeling and thinking positively.

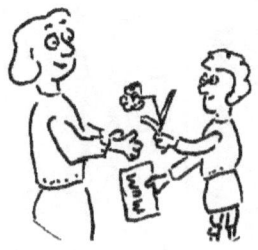

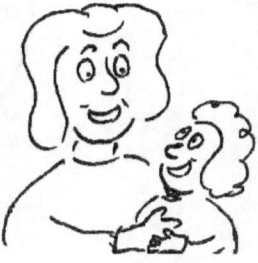

Develop a sense of humour. A joke told in the right way at the right time can help prevent anger.
If we are angry but recognize [by thinking] that something is funny we will feel it is funny.
It is impossible to feel angry,

and acknowledge humour at the same time.

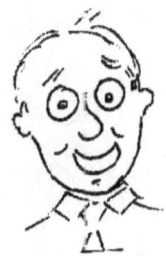

We cannot laugh and be angry at the same time.

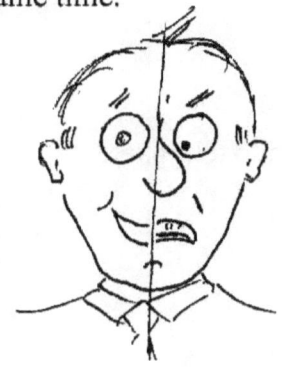

Look to find humour in daily events.

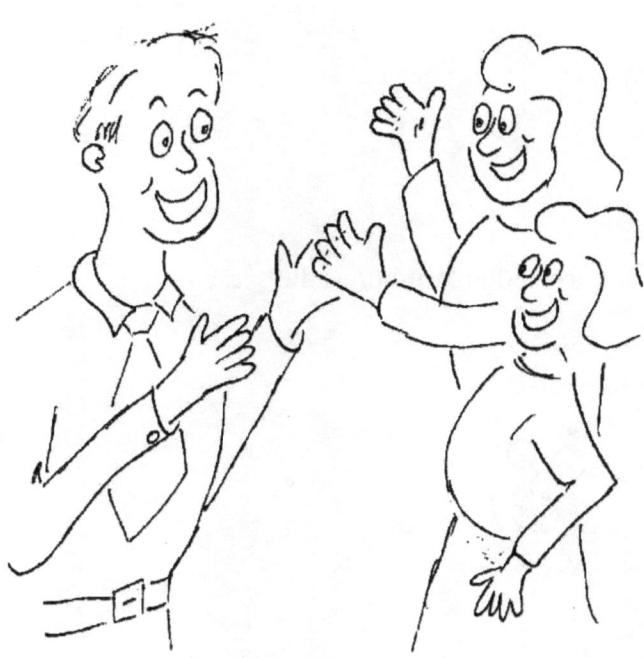

Learn to tell jokes.

Avoid exposure to violence; look for humour instead.

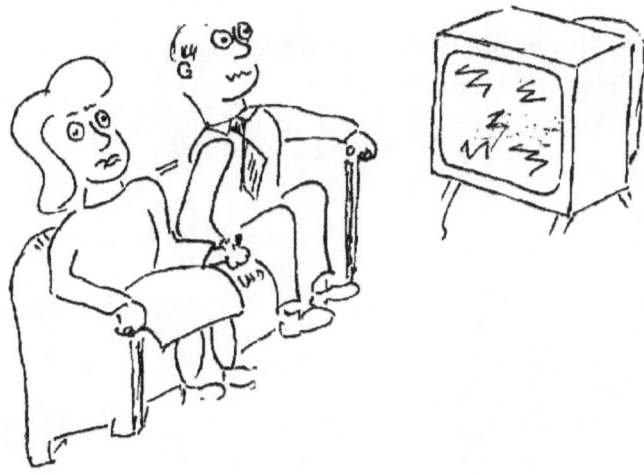

Humour brings relief and relaxation. For a moment we are relieved of our burden of anger.

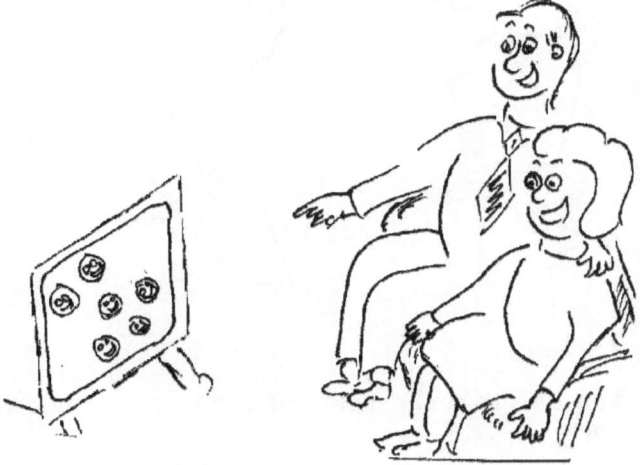

Our A.N.S. activity is reduced.

A SPECIAL CAUSE OF ANGER, Fetal Alcohol Spectrum Disorder (FASD) and other learning disabilities.

Learning disabilities are often a cause of anger.
All our lives we have difficulty.

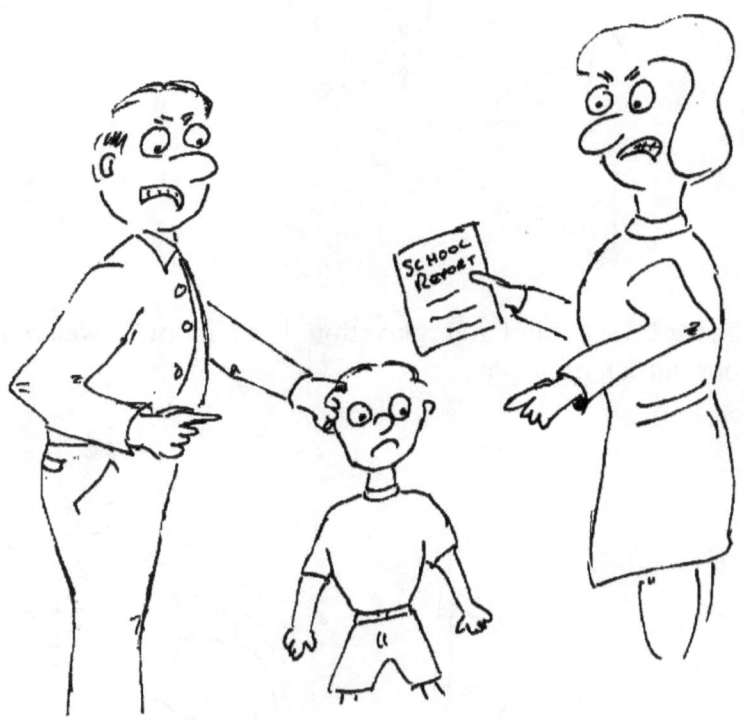

Those who do not understand our problem, become frustrated and angry with us.

Teachers who do not understand our problem,

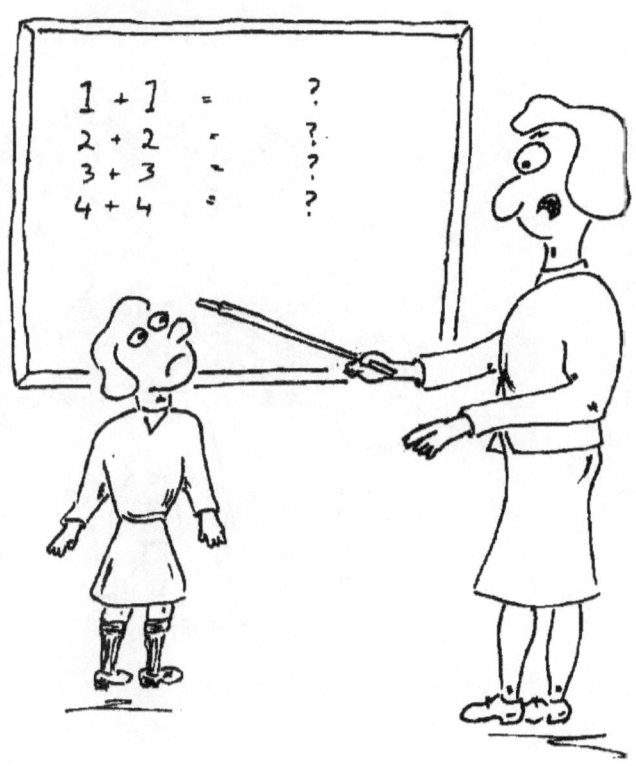

become frustrated and angry with us.

Other children, who do not understand our problem,

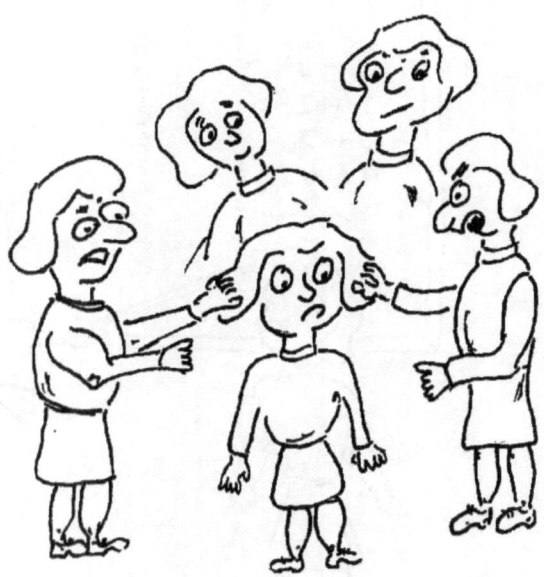

bully, tease, or ignore us.

Co-workers, who do not understand us,

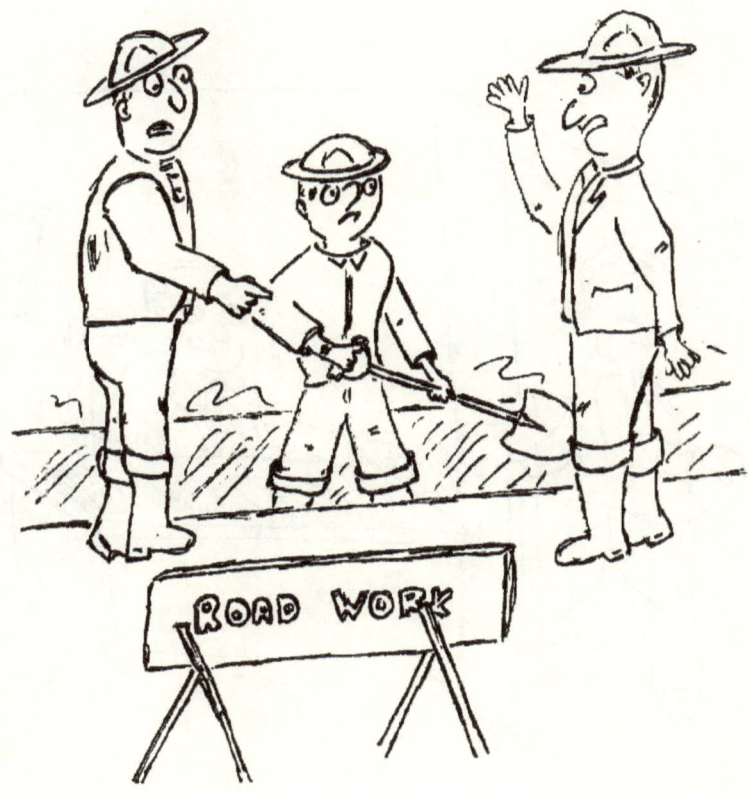

become angry with us.

The boss who does not understand us,

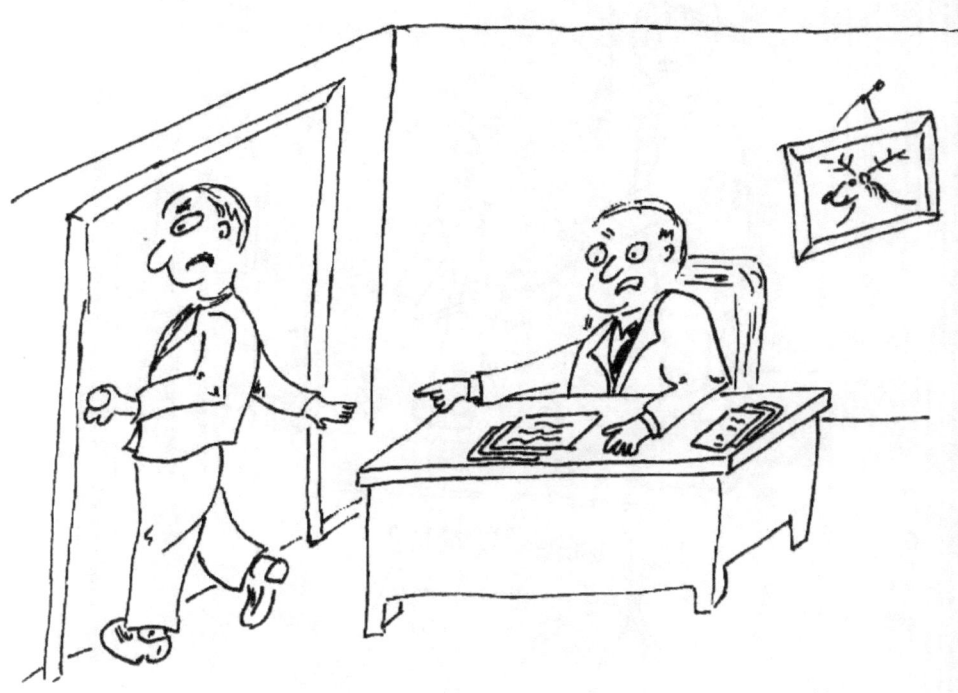

mistreats us, or may fire us.

Because we have poor self-esteem, we continuously feel

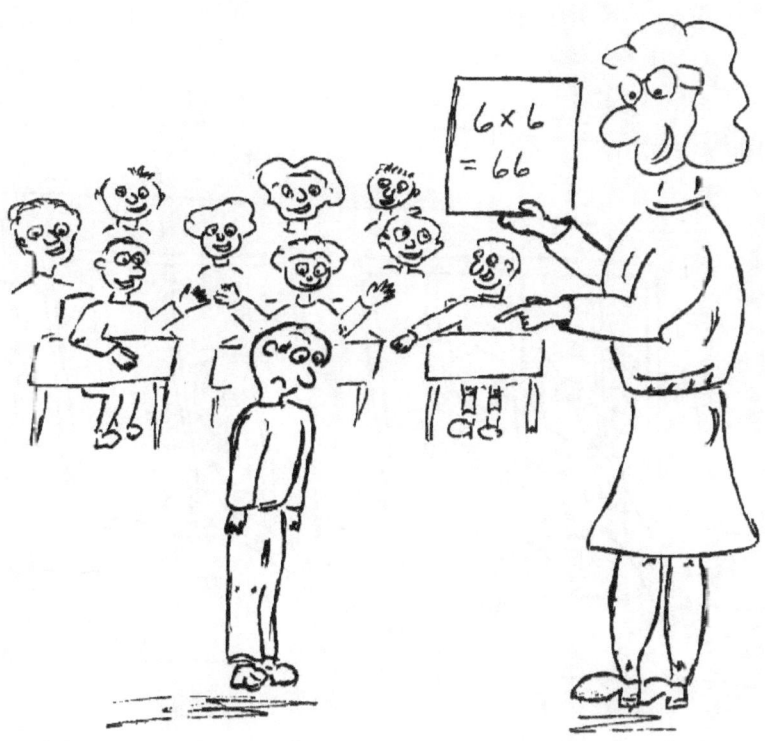

threatened, guilty, ashamed, and angry.

Many of us express our anger outwardly,

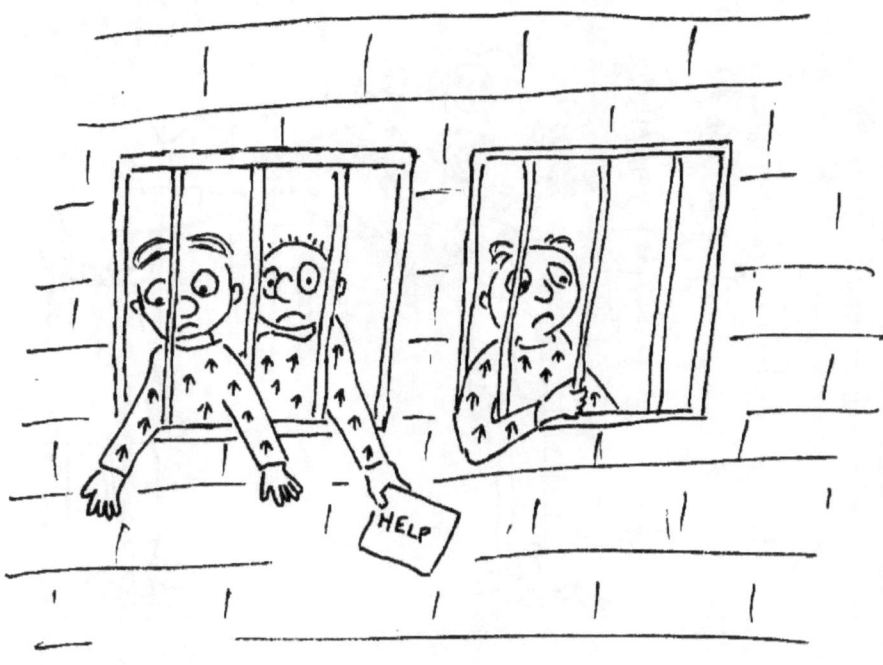

and end up in jail.

Some of us direct our anger inwards

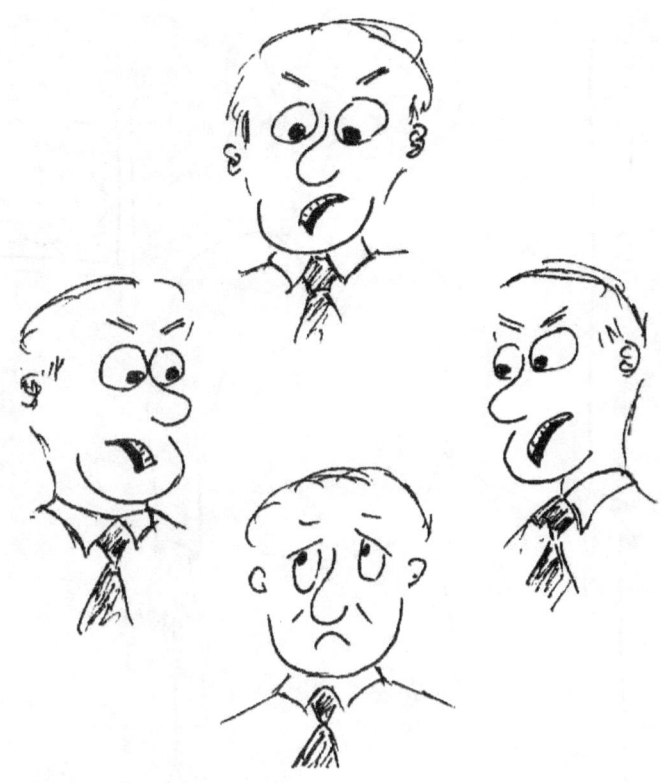

and become depressed.

It is not our fault that we have a learning disability.

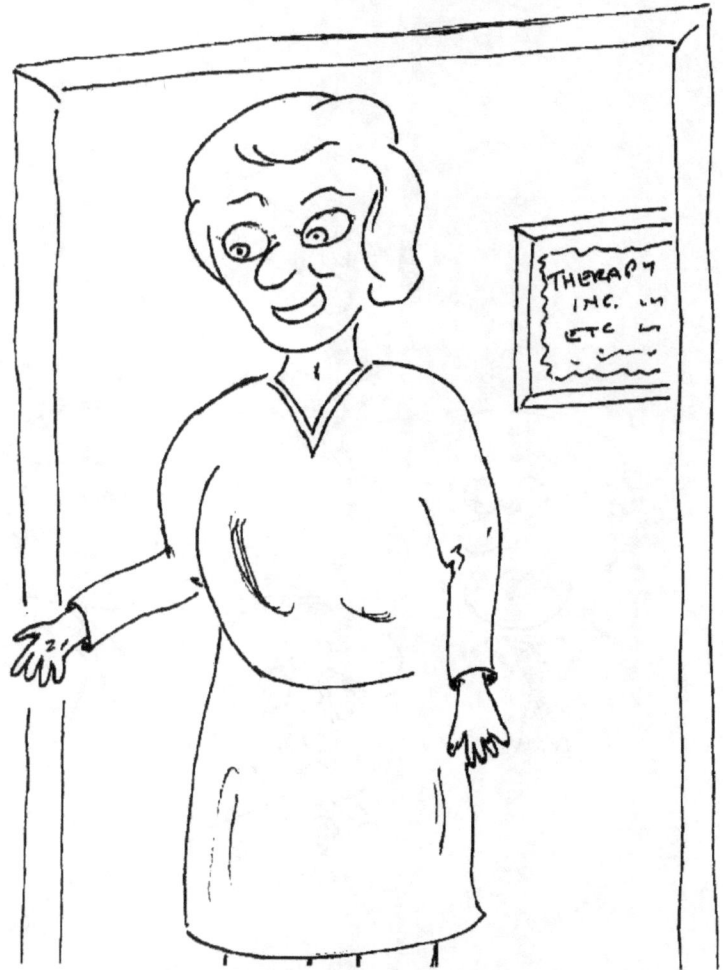

We need to understand that those who hurt us, do so because they do not understand us and are often insecure themselves. Those who are angry with us need to deal with their fear, shame and guilt. This may not be easy. Professional help may be required.

Caregivers need to be educated so that they will understand why we behave differently,

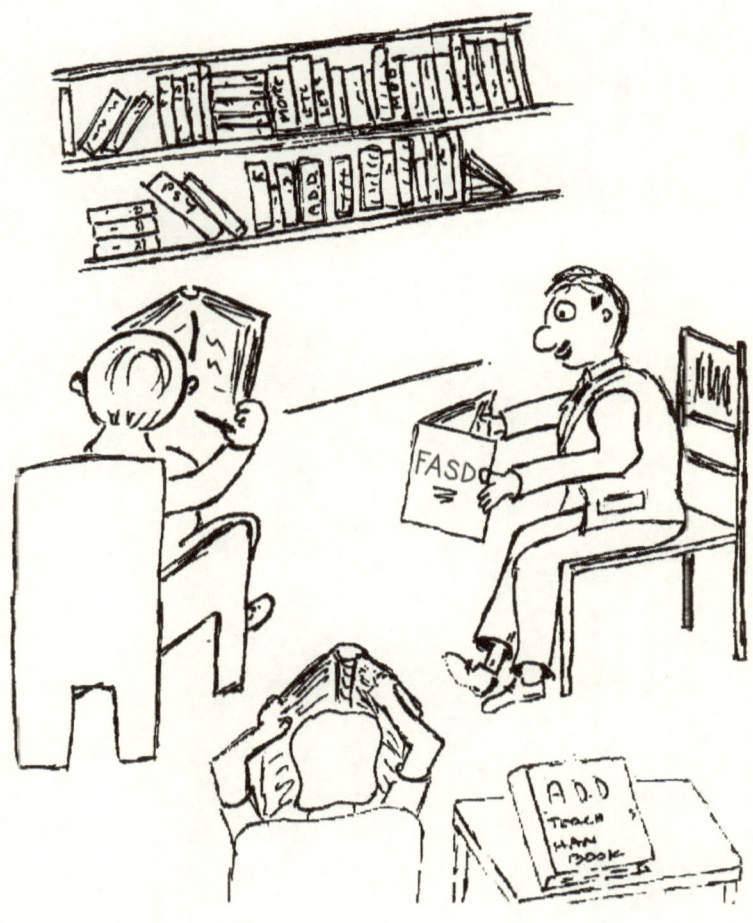

and not become frustrated with us.

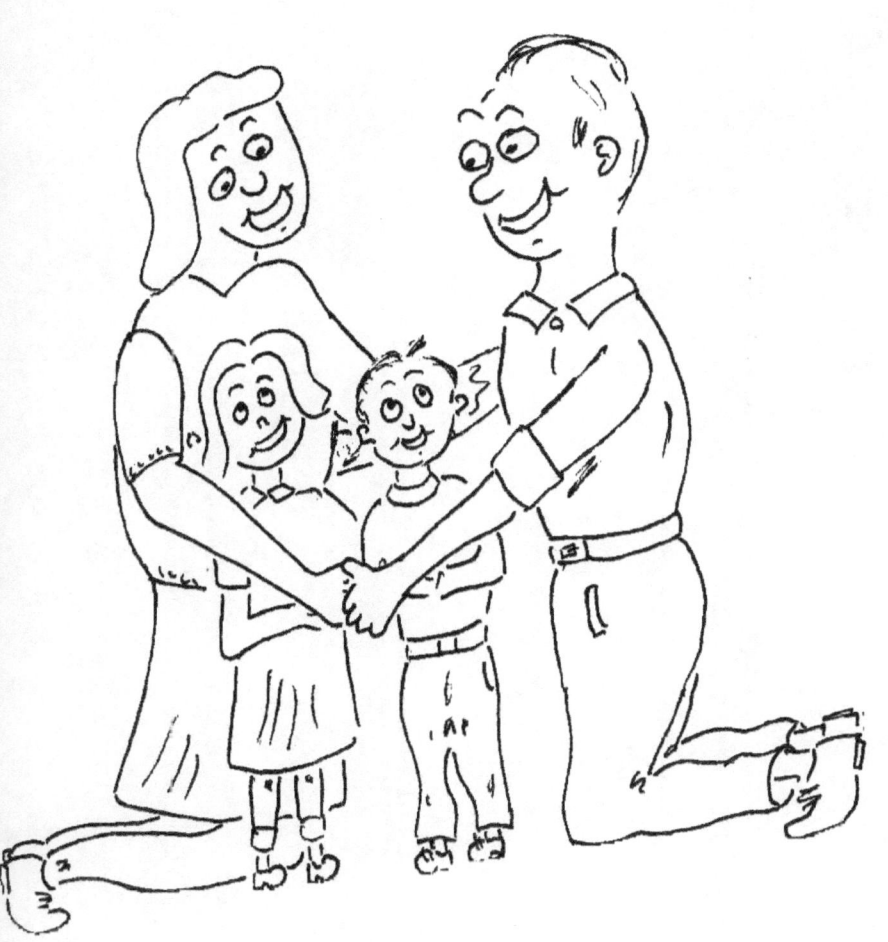

www.ingramcontent.com/pod-product-compliance
Lightning Source LLC
Chambersburg PA
CBHW031252280526
45784CB00004B/1828